THE SEX EDUCATION
ANSWER BOOK

THE SEX EDUCATION ANSWER BOOK

By The Age Responses To Tough Questions
Kids Ask Parents About Sex

by Cath Hakanson

The Sex Education Answer Book: By The Age Responses To Tough Questions
Kids Ask Parents About Sex
by Cath Hakanson

Published by Sex Ed Rescue
PO Box 7903
Cloisters Square WA 6000
Australia
sexedrescue.com

For permission contact:
cath@sexedrescue.com
ISBN-13: 978-0-6487162-0-4

CONTENTS

Introduction

Kids can ask a lot of questions. It's their way of learning about things they don't understand or are curious about.

You just grit your teeth and automatically answer their question in a way that makes sense for them. So, if they ask you why the grass is green, you might say, 'Because I water it each week.' If they were older or wanted more details, you might then start talking about the pigment chlorophyll.

But what if they asked you where babies come from? Or what's a blowjob? Or why are those two men kissing?

Answering those sorts of questions, i.e. the ones about sex, is a lot trickier!

Do you just tell them straight? But what if you give them too much information? Or not enough? And are they old enough, or ready, to hear about this stuff?

Well, you can relax for a moment, because this book will help you with working out how to answer the tough questions that your kids might ask you about sex.

It won't just provide you with age-appropriate answers to your child's questions about sex. It will also help you to understand why you need to answer their questions and how to answer them so that your child knows that they can turn to you for the support, guidance and information that they'll need.

For more than twenty-five years, I've been helping people get more comfortable with sex. I've answered their questions, listened to their fears, empowered them with the right information, and pointed them in the right direction. And after hearing thousands of parents ask me about how to answer their child's questions about sex, I've worked out what they want.

Parents want to know how to have honest conversations about love, sex and relationships that will guide their child, and strengthen their relationship, without feeling embarrassed, awkward or nervous.

But they don't know how to start.

A good place to start is by answering your child's questions about sex. By doing this, you are letting them know that you are a reliable source of information. And as they become teenagers, they will realize that they can talk to you about sex, as well as about other things like drugs, partying and bullying.

This book won't just give you the answers. It will show you how to have the type of relationship with your child where they can talk to you about anything, no matter what. But you need to start talking sooner rather than later, because they are already learning about sex, whether you like it or not!

Empower your child with the right information so that when the time comes, they don't make wrong decisions around love, sex and relationships.

Happy Talking!

Cath

 You can access my FREE sex education course for parents at https://sexedrescue.com/back-to-basics/

HOW TO USE THIS BOOK

Who is this book for?

This book is for parents of children aged between three and fourteen years old.

How does this book work?

There are two parts to this book.

The first part will make sure you get started. It will provide you with all the background information that will help you to answer your child's questions. Don't be tempted to gloss over this section of the book, as it will guide you past the most common parental objections to sex education so that you can get started right away, without any hesitation.

The second part provides the answers. The answers are divided up into each individual age, from the age of three up to fourteen. In each age, you will find the answers to questions that are commonly asked, with extra information for those kids who require more details, practical advice and tips.

How do I use this book to answer my child's questions?

You can use this book to either answer your child's question about sex immediately, or you can delay their answer until later. As you get more comfortable with talking about sex with your child, you will gain enough confidence to start making up your own answers.

Kids don't expect us to know the answer to everything. Plus, they are used to adults turning to the internet, their phone or a book to find information. Which means that they won't think that it is strange that you are looking up the answer to their questions about sex. All your child cares about is getting an answer to their question!

The steps below will outline the steps that you can take to use this book to answer your child's question immediately.

1. Your child asks you a question:
    'What's a blowjob?'

2. Let your child know that you've heard their question:
    'That's a great question. I'm not quite sure, but I'll find out for you now.'

3. Find the answer in the book:
    'Okay, here is the answer. A blowjob is...'

4. Check if they need more information:
    'So, do you have any more questions about what a blowjob is?'

PART 1

GETTING STARTED

Why do kids ask questions about sex?

> Some kids ask lots of questions, and some don't ask many questions at all. Both are perfectly normal!

Children are naturally curious and will usually ask questions about the people and things they hear and see around them. This could be questions like, 'Why does milk come in a carton?', 'Why is the sky blue?', or 'Where do babies come from?'

It is just the way that they make sense of the world around them. And your answers to their questions will satisfy their curiosity and help them to grow and develop in a healthy way.

So, it is very normal for children to ask questions about bodies, babies, pregnancy, families, sexuality and relationships as they grow up.

Why do you need to answer questions about sex?

> Your child will hear about sex regardless of how much you protect them. It is better that they hear about it from you than from someone else.

As exhausting as it can sometimes be, it is important to answer your child's questions about sex, and there are a number of reasons why it is so important.

- You're letting them know that you are a reliable source of information – one that they can keep coming back to for more information.
- Your child will see you as their main source of information. This means they won't need to turn to their friends, the internet or the media for information.
- You'll know that they have accurate facts instead of the misinformation that they will receive from someone or someplace else.
- You can provide them with age-appropriate information that will satisfy their curiosity and allow them to move on to the next great mystery of life.
- You can't stop the negative, highly-sexualized messages that your child will receive about sex from society, but you can counteract them by providing your child with an alternative viewpoint – one that is shaped by sharing your family values about sex.
- You'll be able to satisfy their curiosity about sex, which means that they won't need to look up sexual information online. It is easier for kids to find sexually-explicit information online than it is for them to avoid it!
- Your child will know that if they can talk to you about sex, they can then talk to you about other things, like bullying, inappropriate sexual touch, alcohol and drugs.

How should I answer their questions about sex?

> Don't stress over providing the perfect answer. What really matters is the fact that you are approachable and willing to talk about sex with your child.

There are many different ways to answer your child's questions: simply, with more details, or you can even delay answering them until a better time or place, or until you find the answer.

How you answer depends on how much you know about the subject, your level of confidence and how curious your child is.

For example, if your child asks, 'Where do babies come from?'

Your **simple answer** could be brief and factual: 'Babies come from inside the mother, from a special place called the uterus.' For some kids, this is more than enough information.

But what if that isn't enough information, and they want to know more?

A more **detailed answer** could be: 'Babies come from inside the mother, from a special place called the uterus. A part from the male, called the sperm, and a part from the female, called the ovum or egg, join together to make a baby. The baby then lives inside the uterus, where it grows bigger until it is ready to be born.' You could also read a book together, which would provide your child with more information.

Or you may use a **delayed answer**, if they ask you a question in the wrong place or at the wrong time (like at the table when the in-laws are over for dinner), or if you don't know the answer.

You might say, 'What a great question. How about we talk about that later on?' And, later on, when you have found the answer, or it is a better time to talk, you then provide them with an answer to their earlier question.

If you don't know the answer to their question, then let your child know. You might say, 'I don't know, but how about I find out for you and get back to you with the answer?' Your child will be fine with this, as they are already asking you questions that you can't answer.

Just make sure that you don't forget to follow up with an answer. If you keep on forgetting, or don't get back to them with an answer, eventually your child will stop asking you questions. They will assume that you won't have the answer, or that you aren't comfortable talking about sex with them.

What if they ask a question that isn't age-appropriate?

It is more harmful to ignore your child's questions about sex than it is to answer them.

Sometimes your child might ask you a question that clearly isn't age-appropriate – the sort of question that has your alarm bells ringing and your gut instinct saying, 'Huh, why are they asking about that?'

For example, your child may ask you a question like, 'How do people have sex with dogs?'

Before answering, it is a good idea to find out why they are asking the question with something like, 'Why are you asking about that?'

Then you can work out what sort of response is required.

It is important to remember, though, that kids will often hear about sexual content that is not age-appropriate. They might be watching a movie and hear a sexual reference. Their friend might show them some sexually-explicit images that they found on the internet. Or they might hear giggling at school about licking someone's penis.

When you answer your child's questions about sex, you are telling them that you are askable, and that they can talk to you about anything, no matter what. Which means that when they hear about something that they don't understand, they will ask for your help in making sense of what they have heard.

It is better that your child asks you about how people have sex with dogs than to turn to the internet for that answer. You will provide them with an age-appropriate answer that will satisfy their curiosity. Whereas, by not providing them with an answer, you are igniting their curiosity and giving them no other choice than to search elsewhere for answers. If they type their questions into Google, they will find sexually-explicit images and movies that are highly inappropriate.

Why do I feel so awkward talking about sex with my child?

We all feel awkward talking about sex with kids. But the more you talk, the easier it gets.

You're not alone if the thought of talking about sex with your child makes you feel uncomfortable. We all feel this way at the beginning.

It usually takes a little while to get used to talking about sex with your kids. You will be using words that you may not be used to saying, or talking about stuff that you may not normally talk to your kids (or anyone else) about.

The thing is, though, the more you talk, the easier it gets. Think of it like learning how to ride a bike. When you first get on, you feel quite unsure and clumsy. But the more you practice, the better you get at it. And before you know it, you are confident and riding like a professional!

Sex education is the same. We all feel awkward when we first start talking, but the more you talk, the sooner you start to feel more natural.

It is important to realize, though, that you will never be 100% comfortable with talking to your kids about sex. There will still be times when you feel uncomfortable, no matter how comfortable you think you are with talking about sex.

How can I get more comfortable with talking about sex?

There are a few tricks that can help you with getting more comfortable. And by using this book, you don't have to fumble for the right words.

There are a number of things that you can do that will help you to feel more comfortable with answering your child's questions about sex.

ACTIVITY: FAMILIARIZE YOURSELF WITH THE ANSWERS

Before you even think of using them to answer your child's questions, you need to go and have a good look at the answers. So, go and look at the answers for your child's age.

Get familiar with what you could be talking about to a child of that age, and how it is said.

And don't be tempted to look at scripts for older kids – you will just end up feeling overwhelmed!

ACTIVITY: FAMILIARIZE YOURSELF WITH THE WORDS

Sometimes we can feel uncomfortable just saying words like 'penis' and 'vulva.' They may be words that we just aren't used to saying, or we may have been taught that they were words that shouldn't be said in public.

If you can't say sexual words, you will struggle with talking to your kids about sex.

So, we need to look at finding a way to get you more comfortable with using these words.

This activity will help you to begin to feel more comfortable with saying sex words and using them with your child.

This what I want you to do:

1. Stand in front of your bathroom mirror alone.
2. Say the following words aloud:
   clitoris, vagina, vulva, cervix, urethra, uterus, ovary, ovum, fallopian tubes, anus, scrotum, testicles, penis, foreskin, sperm, semen, ejaculation, erection, orgasm, lubrication, menstruation, periods, sex, sexual intercourse, pornography, porn, oral sex, anal sex.
3. Pay attention to your reaction. Did you flinch or squirm when saying these words aloud?
4. Repeat this list of words daily until you begin to feel more comfortable when saying the words.

Then you can start to use these words in your everyday conversations with your child.

Start looking for opportunities to use words like penis, vulva, breasts, or puberty.

You could use them at bath time, when getting dressed, when playing games (e.g., where's your nose, where's your penis, where's your...)

ACTIVITY: FAMILIARIZE YOURSELF WITH THE ANSWERS

When you are comfortable with saying the words, you can move on to this activity, where you will now start to get more comfortable with answering your child's questions.

This what I want you to do:

1. Select one or two answers from the book for your child's age.
2. Read these answers aloud for a minute or two.
3. Pay attention to your reaction. Did you flinch or squirm when saying these words aloud?
4. Practice saying the same scripts aloud a dozen or more times each, until you feel more comfortable saying these words out loud. Then

try some different scripts and practice saying them aloud until you are comfortable with saying them.

When you are comfortable with saying them aloud to yourself, you could then move on to saying them with a partner or a friend, and then your children.

But what if I've never talked to my child about sex before?

The first conversation is always the hardest!

So, what do you do if this is the first time that you have ever talked about sex with your child?

The best way to get started is to warn your child that you are going to start talking about sex.

First, let your child know that you are ready to start talking about sex. You could try explaining that you have realized that you haven't talked about sex before, but that you would like to change that.

You could try saying something like, 'I watched an interesting show on TV last night (heard an interview on the radio/ read a good book/ was talking with a friend/ attended a workshop), and they talked about how important it is for parents to talk about sex with their children. It made me realize that sex is something that we haven't talked about before.'

Second, explain why you haven't talked to them about sex before. You could say:

- 'It's something that my parents didn't talk about very much when I was a kid, either.'
- 'I've always been worried that I would be bringing it up at the wrong time or the wrong place.'
- 'I've always worried that I would get it all wrong or do as bad a job as my parents did.'

- 'I've always been worried about either saying too much or too little, or even the wrong thing.'
- 'Talking about sex makes me feel really uncomfortable.'

Third, explain what is going to change.

You could try saying, 'I want us to be able to talk about anything, including sex. So, you are going to hear me start talking about love, sex and relationships. If you have any questions or want to talk about something, I want you to know that I am always available.'

But is my child ready to hear about sex?

'I know that I need to talk to my kids about sex, but I still worry about whether I am doing the right thing or not.'

Sometimes it can feel as if there are more reasons not to talk than there are to talk.

Maybe you just find talking about sex way too embarrassing. Well, you're not alone if you do because we all feel awkward when we first start talking about sex with our kids. But the more you talk, the sooner you start to feel more natural and less embarrassed.[1]

Maybe you feel that your child is too young to be hearing about sex. Maybe they are, and maybe they aren't. But they are going to hear about sex regardless, so isn't it better that they hear about it from you, so that you can provide them with the facts before they get misinformation from someone or someplace else?[2]

---

1 Dyson, Sue. (2010). *Parents and Sex Education. A consultation with parents on educating their children about sexual health at home and school.* Western Australia. Dept. of Health - Public Health Division. La Trobe University - Australian Research Centre in Sex, Health, and Society. Accessed 3 November 2017 http://healthywa.wa.gov.au/~/media/Files/HealthyWA/Original/ Sexual-health/report_sex_ed_and_parents_consultation.pdf

2 Dyson, Sue. (2010). Parents and Sex Education. Parents' attitudes to sexual health education in WA schools. Western Australia. Dept. of Health - Public Health Division. La Trobe University - Australian Research Centre in Sex, Health, and Society. Accessed 3 November 2017 http://healthywa.wa.gov.au/~/media/Files/HealthyWA/Original/Sexual-health/Sexual healthParentsShortReport.pdf

Maybe you're worried that by talking about sex with your child, that you will be sexualizing them? Or giving them permission to be sexually active? There is a lot of research that tells us that you won't be[3],[4]. Sex education means that your child is more likely to delay sex, to have fewer sexual partners, and to use contraception.[5]

Maybe you're worried that you will give your child too much information. Don't be, as kids only take in as much information as they are able to understand. If you give them too much information, they will just become bored and stop listening.[6]

Maybe you think your child doesn't want to hear about sex from you. Well, you're wrong. Research tells us that teenagers consistently say their parents are the most important influence when it comes to making decisions about sex, even more than their friends, the media, religious leaders, their brothers or sisters, or their teachers. Parental influence does decline as kids get older, though, which means that it is important to start talking sooner rather than later.[7]

What sexual values and beliefs do I share with my child?

What sexual attitudes and behaviors are okay (and not okay) in your family?

This is the time your child will be working out their own thoughts, beliefs and attitudes about the world around them. They will be making important

---

3 SRE – The evidence (2015) Sex Education Forum Evidence Briefing. Published by the NCB (National Children's Bureau) Accessed 3 November 2017 http://www.sexeducationforum.org.uk/media/28306/SRE-the-evidence-March-2015.pdf

4 Kirby, D. (2007). Emerging Answers 2007: New Research Findings on Programs to Reduce Teen Pregnancy —Full Report. Washington, DC: The National Campaign to Prevent Teen and Unplanned Pregnancy. Accessed 3 November 2017 https://thenationalcampaign.org/resource/emerging-answers-2007%E2%80%94full-report

5 Albert, B. (2012). With One Voice 2012: America's Adults and Teens Sound Off About Teen Pregnancy. Washington, DC: The National Campaign to Prevent Teen and Unplanned Pregnancy. Accessed 3 November 2017 https://thenationalcampaign.org/resource/one-voice-2012

6 Goldman, R. & J. (1988) Show me yours! Understanding Children's Sexuality. Australia. Ringwood.

7 The National Campaign to Prevent Teen and Unplanned Pregnancy. (2016). Survey Says: Parent Power Washington, DC: Author. Accessed 3 November 2017 https://thenationalcampaign.org/resource/survey-says-october-2016

decisions about what attitudes and behaviors are okay, and not okay, when it comes to love, sex and relationships. This is why it is so important that you are there to guide them. You can't tell your child what their values and beliefs will be; you can only guide them.

Do you have the exact same values as your parents? Probably not. You may share some of the same values as your parents, but you will also have some that are yours alone. And your siblings will have a completely different set of values too, despite the fact that you were all influenced by your parents in the same way. The reason that you share some of the same values as your parents is because they influenced you. Some of their values must have made sense, and you took them on board as your own. And some you developed by yourself, influenced by what you saw on TV, heard in music, or learned by talking with your friends and by watching your peers.

Your child will be the same. They will make up their own set of values, but they will listen to what you say. If you don't share your values with your child, you can't expect to have any influence on what sexual attitudes and behaviors they develop. If you want to have any say in it, you will have to talk to them and explain why you feel the way you do.

Let's use contraception as an example:

Don't just talk about the fact that you can prevent pregnancies with contraception. Share with your child what your thoughts are about contraception and unplanned pregnancy. Explain the reasons behind your belief so that your child understands why. By sharing your values with your child, you are providing them with a moral compass to guide them as they make sense of the mixed messages that they will receive from the media, their peers, and the world around them.

Questions to ask your child

Here are some questions or comments that you can use with your child that will help to turn a simple question into a more meaningful conversation:

- What do you think?
- What do you feel?
- What feels right to you?
- That's a good point.
- I disagree, but I see your point.
- How do you think that happens?
- Why are you asking?
- Tell me some more.
- Hmm ... what do you mean by that?
- How do you want to deal with it?
- Where did you hear that?

Tips for answering your child's questions

Now, before you even think about answering your child's questions about sex, there are some principles that will help to make your conversations more successful:

- Try to answer questions straight away, i.e. as soon as possible. If you can't, make sure you get back to them with an answer later on (and don't forget).
- Find out what your child knows first by asking, 'What do you think?' This way, you'll know how much they already know. Plus, you'll know exactly what it is that they are asking!
- Keep it super simple. Use basic, clear language. Try to keep your answers to responses of one-or-two sentences. Then, if they want more information, provide it.
- Check that your child understood what you said by asking, 'So, did that answer your question?' or, 'Does that make sense to you?'
- Ask if they have any more questions.

- Tell them when you don't know the answer. Say, 'I don't know,' find the answer, and get back to them with it. Don't lie or tell them things that aren't true.
- Share your values and beliefs – remember to tell them what sexual behaviors and attitudes are okay (and not okay) in your family, and why.
- Try to use the correct terms. It is okay to use some cute names, but only if they know the correct name as well.
- Use your everyday voice – the one you normally use when you answer their questions.
- Embarrassment comes with the territory! The more you talk, the easier it gets!
- Don't worry about giving them too much information. If kids don't understand something, they promptly forget whatever it is that you just said to them.
- It is many small conversations over time, so don't feel that you have to cover it all at once. You have years to talk about this stuff!

Books

Books make sex education a lot easier, mainly because they contain the facts that you don't need to remember.

You can find up-to-date lists of age-specific sex education books here - **https://sexedrescue.com/sex-education-books-for-children/**

Also, don't forget about your local library. If they don't stock the book you want, request it as it will help other parents too!

 You can access my FREE sex education course for parents at https://sexedrescue.com/back-to-basics/

THE BODY PARTS

When you start talking about sex, it is important to know the names of the different parts you will be talking about. Below you will find some images and child-friendly definitions that both you and your child will understand.

And if you are unsure about how to say any of these words, use an **online dictionary** for the pronunciation.

Before you use these words with your child, first practice saying them aloud to yourself. Talking about sex can be stressful enough without the added worry of trying to remember how to pronounce the words correctly!

Female Parts

Anus: The opening that is below the vulva, where feces (poo) comes out. Males have an anus too.

Bladder: A stretchy bag that holds the urine (pee) before it comes out of the body. The urine leaves the bladder through a small tube called the urethra. Males have a bladder too.

Cervix: The opening of the uterus that joins it with the vagina. You can find it deep inside, at the very top of your vagina.

Clitoris: A part that is behind the vulva and wraps around the vagina. The smallest part, about the size of a pea, can be seen outside the body, hidden under a small bump of skin, just above the urethra where the pee comes out. It can feel good when you touch it.

Fallopian tubes: Special tubes, like cooked spaghetti, that carry the egg from the ovaries to the uterus.

Labia majora: The outer lips that surround the vaginal opening. These are thicker and will eventually be covered in hair on the outside skin.

Labia minora: The inner lips that surround the vaginal opening. These are thinner and will not be covered in hair.

Mons pubis: The soft rounded area that sits above the pubic bone. Eventually, it will be covered in pubic hair.

Ovaries: Special organs that produce the eggs or ova. They are about the size of a grape.

Rectum: A tube that is used to store feces (poo) before it is pushed out through the anus. Males have a rectum too.

Uterus: A bag made of muscle that is about the size of a pear. It is the place for a baby to grow, and stretches bigger as the baby grows.

Urethra: A narrow tube that leaves from the bladder and comes out of a small opening in the vulva.

Urethral opening: The small opening in the vulva where the urethra comes out of the body. It can be found between the clitoris and the vagina. Males have a urethral opening too.

Vagina: A stretchy tube that goes from the uterus to the outside of the body. It is the opening that you can feel at the bottom of the vulva.

Vulva: Thick folds of skin that cover the opening to the vagina. There is an outer part, which is the labia majora, and an inner part, which is the labia minora.

FEMALE
INTERNAL (FRONT VIEW)

FALLOPIAN TUBES

UTERUS

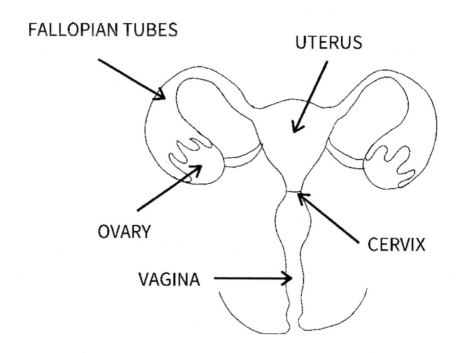

OVARY

CERVIX

VAGINA

FEMALE
INTERNAL (SIDE VIEW)

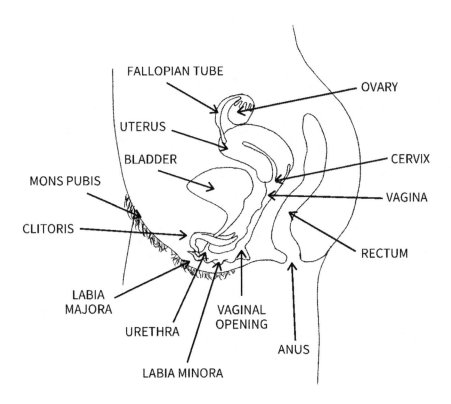

CLITORIS

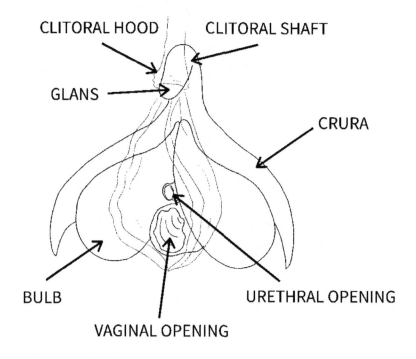

CLITORAL HOOD

CLITORAL SHAFT

GLANS

CRURA

BULB

URETHRAL OPENING

VAGINAL OPENING

FEMALE
EXTERNAL

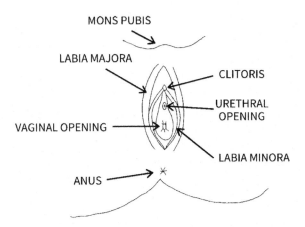

MONS PUBIS

LABIA MAJORA

CLITORIS

URETHRAL OPENING

VAGINAL OPENING

LABIA MINORA

ANUS

Male Parts

Anus: The opening that is behind the scrotum, where feces (poo) comes out. Females have an anus too.

Bladder: A stretchy bag that holds the urine (pee) before it comes out of the body. The urine leaves the bladder through a small tube called the urethra. Females have a bladder too.

Corona: The ridge that runs around the bottom of the glans, where it joins the body of the penis.

Cowper's gland: These two small, round glands (the size of a pea) are found underneath the prostate gland. When a male starts to feel sexually aroused, they will start to make a special fluid that will lubricate the penis and keep the sperm safe as it travels through the urethra. The other name for this part is the bulbourethral gland.

Epididymis: The testicle is connected to the epididymis. Once sperm has been made in the testicles, it is sent to the epididymis. It is here that the sperm is grown up or matured, ready for reproduction. If felt through the scrotum, it will feel soft and squishy, like a piece of cooked spiral pasta.

Foreskin: The loose skin at the end of the penis. It protects the end of the penis, the glans, which is very sensitive to touch.

Frenulum: A sensitive piece of skin on the underside of the penis where the foreskin attaches itself to the glans. It helps the foreskin to contract or shrink itself over the glans and can only be seen when the foreskin is fully retracted.

Glans: The head or the tip of the penis. It has many nerve endings, which means it is sensitive to touch. In uncircumcised penises, this will be covered by the foreskin.

Penis: The part that hangs in front of the scrotum and sticks out. Urine comes out of the small opening at the end of it. The penis is also used for sexual intercourse, where it becomes erect, and semen comes out of the end of it, through the urethral opening.

Prostate gland: A gland that is at the base of the penis, near the bladder. The urethra runs through the center of it. The prostate gland helps with bladder control and secretes fluids that mix with the sperm to make semen.

Scrotum: The soft bag of squishy skin between the legs that holds and protects the testicles. It has a muscle that makes it expand with heat (e.g. when having a warm bath) and shrink with cold (e.g. when swimming in the ocean). This keeps the testicles at the right temperature to protect the sperm.

Seminal vesicles: A pair of glands that lie on either side of the bladder. They open into the vas deferens and secrete fluids that mix with the sperm to make semen.

Shaft: The length or body of the penis.

Testicles: The male sex organs that make sperm. They are two soft oval shaped parts that will grow much bigger during puberty, to about the size of a plum. Sperm is made in the testicles. If felt through the scrotum, a testicle will feel like a hard-boiled egg that has been peeled.

Urethra: A narrow tube that leaves from the bladder, and goes through the penis to the small opening at the tip of the penis (urethral opening). It also carries the semen after it leaves the vas deferens.

Urethral opening: The slit at the end of the penis (through the glans) where urine and semen come out. Females have a urethral opening too.

Vas deferens: The tube that connects the testicles/epididymis to the prostate and seminal vesicles. If felt through the scrotum, it will feel like a piece of cooked spaghetti.

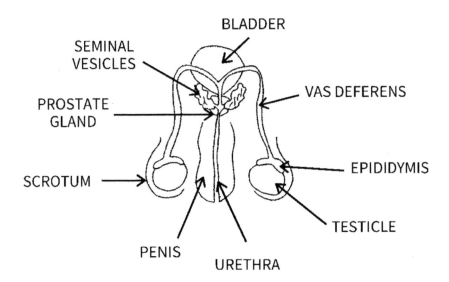

MALE
INTERNAL (FRONT VIEW)

BLADDER

SEMINAL VESICLES

VAS DEFERENS

PROSTATE GLAND

SCROTUM

EPIDIDYMIS

TESTICLE

PENIS

URETHRA

MALE
INTERNAL (SIDE VIEW)

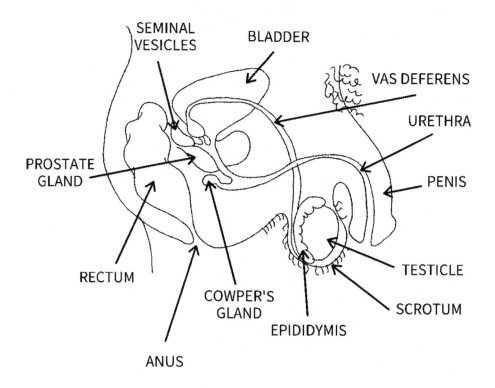

MALE
EXTERNAL (INTACT)

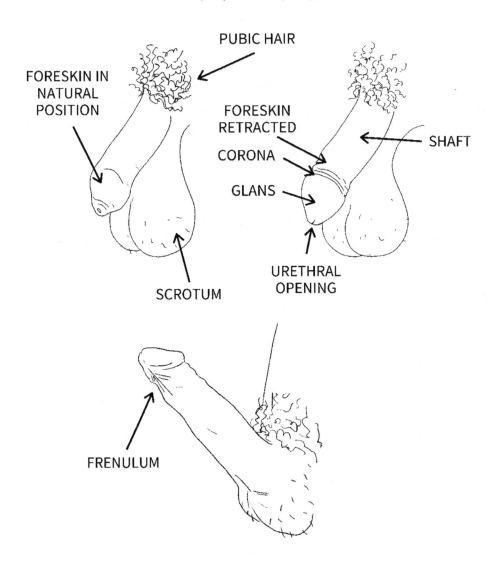

PUBIC HAIR

FORESKIN IN
NATURAL
POSITION

FORESKIN
RETRACTED

CORONA

GLANS

SHAFT

URETHRAL
OPENING

SCROTUM

FRENULUM

MALE
EXTERNAL (CIRCUMCISED)

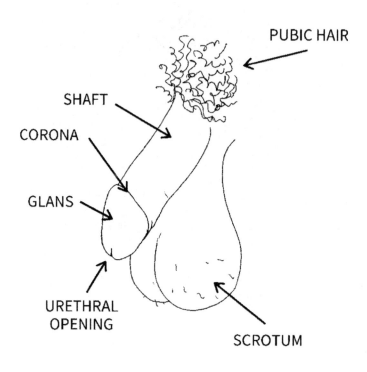

PUBIC HAIR

SHAFT

CORONA

GLANS

URETHRAL
OPENING

SCROTUM

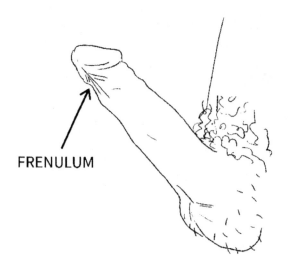

FRENULUM

CHILD SEXUAL DEVELOPMENT

So, what does healthy sexual development in your child look like? Keep in mind that some kids develop faster or slower than others, and may not display all of these behaviors.

Don't be surprised if your child reflects behavior that is a year or two older or younger than their age. As you know, every kid is different and is developing on their own schedule.

And if you are ever unsure about any sexual behavior in your child, the first place to go is the Traffic lights app (http://www.true.org.au/Education/traffic-lights). This low-priced app will help you work out whether you should worry or not, and how best to manage the behavior.

THREE YEAR OLDS

Three is the age where they are usually pretty curious about their own body and everybody else's! They will want to know the names of all their parts (genitals included) and openly talk about where pee and poo come from. They will also work out that touching their own genitals can feel nice, and will happily do this at any time or place, regardless of who else is around. They are now becoming aware of gender differences and may start to 'play doctor,' where they are trying to work out if their friends' genitals are different from theirs. They will also be starting to identify as a particular gender, i.e. male, female, both or neither. Some may start to become curious about where babies come from, especially if there is a sibling on the way. Or pretend that they have a baby growing in their belly.

FOUR YEAR OLDS

Four is the age where they start to ask questions about where babies come from and how they grow. It is more of a curiosity about how they got here than an interest in sexual intercourse. They are still pretty curious about their own body, and usually yours as well. They might start to ask questions like, 'Why do you have hair?' or 'Why don't you have a penis?' They will know the names of all of their body parts (genitals included) and openly talk about them, as well as where pee and poo come from. They may have discovered that touching their own genitals can feel nice or relax them, and will happily do this at any time or place, regardless of who else is around. They are usually aware of gender differences and may start to 'play doctor,' where they are trying to work out the differences between males and females. They will also be starting to identify as a particular gender, i.e. male, female, both or neither. You will see this in their play and in what they say.

FIVE YEAR OLDS

Five is the age where they are still curious about pregnancy and where babies come from, but they may now be wanting to know a few more details, like how babies are made. They may still be curious about bodies and may still ask questions like, 'Why do you have hair?' or, 'Why don't you have a penis?' They will know the names of all of their body parts (genitals included) and may still openly talk about them, as well as where pee and poop come from. They may have discovered that touching their own genitals can feel nice or can relax them, but are starting to understand that there is a time and a place for it. They are now aware of gender differences and may start to 'play doctor,' where they are trying to work out the differences between males and females. They will also be starting to identify as a particular gender, i.e. male, female, both or neither. You will see this in their play and in what they say.

SIX YEAR OLDS

Six is the age where they usually know about where babies come from, how they are made and how they get out, but they won't be as interested in it as they were before. They may still be curious about bodies, will know the names of their genitals, and may enjoy 'toilet talk,' i.e. using words like poo and bum a lot!

They may also start to become shy about their body and even demand privacy at times. They may still touch their genitals (masturbate) and 'play doctor' (look at their playmates' genitals) but will now start to hide it from you. By now, they are usually well aware of gender differences and will start to behave in a gender-specific way, picking up on messages as to how they are expected to behave.

SEVEN YEAR OLDS

Seven is the age where they're still curious about how babies are made and born, and will think that sexual intercourse is funny or a strange thing to do. They will mainly play with same-sex friends and may be teased if they don't behave in their pre-defined gender role (e.g. boys will be teased for liking the color pink). When playing, though, they are usually still happy to role-play as someone of the opposite sex (e.g. females may pretend to be the daddy). You may find that they come home from school asking questions about sexual things that they have heard other kids talking about. If they touch their genitals (masturbate) or 'play doctor' (look at their playmates' genitals), it is now more likely to be hidden. They may also become shy about their body and want more privacy. 'Toilet talk' is common, i.e. using words like poo and bum a lot!

EIGHT YEAR OLDS

Eight is the age where they're curious about sex, but they still see it as a funny or strange thing to do. They will mainly play with same-sex friends and may be teased if they don't behave in their pre-defined gender role (e.g. boys will be teased for liking the color pink). You may find that they come home from school asking questions about sexual things that they have heard other kids talking about. Touching their genitals (masturbation) will be hidden. They may also become shy about their body and want more privacy. 'Toilet talk' is still common, i.e. using words like poo and bum a lot! Some children may start to show the first signs of puberty, like moodiness.

NINE YEAR OLDS

Nine is the age where they may be talking about sex with their friends or looking for the answers to their questions themselves, online or through books. So, the chances of them stumbling across content that is *not* age-appropriate is very high. They may also be starting to connect with their peers and strangers online through messaging, chatrooms and social media while using mobile devices (phones, music, tablets) and computers. If they masturbate, it will be hidden. They may be shy about their body and want more privacy. Some kids may be starting to show the first signs of puberty. If you're lucky, they will slowly be outgrowing 'toilet talk,' i.e. using words like poo and bum a lot!

TEN YEAR OLDS

Ten is the age where they are starting to grow up. They may be a lot more aware of how they look and may even begin to question if their body is normal, especially if the first signs of puberty are beginning to appear. For males, the first signs of puberty are usually a few years later than they are for females. They are now beginning to play with both boys and girls, with some even becoming interested in love and romance for the first time. If they masturbate, it will be hidden. They may be shy about their body and want more privacy. They may now feel embarrassed to talk about sex with their parents, which means that they will talk with friends instead, or look for information online or in books. The chances of them stumbling across content that is *not* age-appropriate is very high.

ELEVEN YEAR OLDS

Eleven is the age where the first signs of puberty may be showing; it's usually a few years earlier in females than it is for males. They may be concerned about their changing body and compare themselves to their peers, wondering if they're normal or not. The desire to fit in with their peers is growing stronger, and they don't want to be different, left out or seen to be abnormal. Some may start to become interested in love and romance, and may experience sexual feelings for the first time. As they become aware of these feelings, they may now masturbate for pleasure. They may be shy about their body and want more privacy. They may now feel embarrassed to talk about sex with their parents, which means that they will talk with friends instead or look for information online or in books. The chances of them stumbling across content that is *not* age-appropriate is very high. They may also be connecting with their peers and strangers online through messaging, chatrooms and social media while using mobile devices (phones, music, tablets) and computers.

TWELVE YEAR OLDS

Twelve is the age where many will be showing some physical signs of puberty and some females may have their first menstrual period. If they are yet to change, they will be aware of their friends' changing bodies and will begin to wonder if they are normal, and when their body, too, will start to change. Some may start to become interested in love and romance and may experience sexual feelings for the first time. As they become aware of these feelings, they may now masturbate for pleasure. They may be shy about their body and want more privacy. It is now that they begin to show an interest in sexual topics. They may now feel embarrassed to talk about sex with their parents, which means that they will talk with friends instead or look for information in books or view sexually-explicit images and videos. They may also be connecting with their peers and strangers online through messaging, chatrooms and social media while using mobile devices (phones, music, tablets) and computers.

THIRTEEN YEAR OLDS

Thirteen is the age where they are beginning to look more like an adult than a child, but they do not have the emotional maturity of an adult. Their bodies will be changing due to puberty, and they may now be capable of reproducing (becoming a parent). Females may have had their first menstrual period, while some boys may now begin to ejaculate semen. Some may start to become interested in sex, and may experience sexual feelings for the first time. As they become aware of these feelings, they may now masturbate for pleasure. If they have a romantic relationship, it is more social and experimental, and short-lived. Some may know which sex they are attracted to. Peer influence is strong, and they are concerned about what others think of them. They are likely to be shy about their body and want more privacy. They may feel embarrassed to talk about sex with their parents, which means that they will talk with friends instead or look for information in books or view sexually-explicit images and videos. They may also be connecting with their peers and strangers online through messaging, chatrooms and social media while using mobile devices (phones, music, tablets) and computers.

FOURTEEN YEAR OLDS

Fourteen is the age where they are a lot more mature and aware of their sexuality. Puberty will still be changing their body, and they will now be capable of reproducing (becoming a parent). This doesn't mean, though, that they are emotionally ready for parenting. Their new sexual feelings are usually limited to masturbation, but may lead to flirting, hugging and kissing. If they have a romantic relationship, it is more social and experimental than sexual. They will usually know their sexual orientation (which gender they are attracted to) but may still be working it out. It isn't uncommon for them to be attracted to someone of the same sex, but this does not necessarily reflect their sexual orientation. Peer influence is not as strong as it was before. They are likely to be shy about their body and want more privacy. They may feel embarrassed to talk about sex with their parents, which means that they will talk with friends instead or look for information in books or view sexually-explicit images and videos. They may also be connecting with their peers and strangers online through messaging, chatrooms and social media while using mobile devices (phones, music, tablets) and computers.

PART 2

THE ANSWERS

Every child is different. Some will have lots of questions, and some won't. And some children will be more curious about sexuality than others – all is normal!

If the content seems 'too mature' for your child, go back a year and use that content. If your child wants to know more, they'll let you know by asking more questions.

When answering your child's questions, don't forget to:

- Find out what your child knows first by asking, 'What do you think?' This way you'll know how much they already know. Plus, you'll know exactly what it is that they are asking!
- Check that your child understood what you said by asking, 'So, did that answer your question?' or, 'Does that make sense to you?'
- Ask if they have any more questions.
- You will find extra information available for some questions, just in case you have a child who wants to know more! Provide it if your child asks or if you feel comfortable sharing it.

And don't forget that there are many different ways to answer your child's questions about sex. This book just provides you with some of the different types of answers. And if you mess it up the first time, that's fine, as you will have plenty more opportunities to try again.

3 YEAR OLDS

Babies (and where they come from)

Where do babies come from?

They don't want to know about sex. They just want to know where they were before they were born.

Babies come from inside the mommy, near the belly.

EXTRA INFO: Babies grow in a special place near the mommy's belly. It is called the uterus.

Where does the baby grow?

The baby grows inside a special bag that is near the mommy's belly.

EXTRA INFO: The proper name for this place is the uterus.

How are babies made?

To make a baby, you need a part from a male and a part from a female.

EXTRA INFO: The special parts are called cells (or the egg and sperm).

Can we have a new baby?

Keep your answer simple. They don't need to know why!

45

Yes	No	Maybe

Can I have a baby?

No, not yet. Only adults can have babies.

Bodies

Learn more about teaching your child the names of their genitals in this article — https://sexedrescue.com/naming-private-parts/. You can find child-friendly diagrams to show your child here - https://sexedrescue.com/products/. And you can find books for talking to your child about their body here - https://sexedrescue.com/childrens-books-about-private-parts/.

What's this part called?

Just name the body part in your normal everyday voice. You can start off with penis and scrotum (or testicles) or vulva and vagina. You can add in the other parts (foreskin, urethra, clitoris) if you want or name then when your child asks or as they get older. Try to keep it simple!

That's called a …

Why does my penis go hard? (erection)

You can let them know that erections have a sexual purpose when they are a bit older and curious about sexual intercourse. At the moment, though, it is just an amazing thing that their body can do.

That is what penises can do.

EXTRA INFO: It is called an erection.

Why don't I have a penis (or vulva)?

Today, we are aware that gender (boy or girl) does not always match your sex (male or female). Some children are intersex (their genitals do not look male or female) or they may have a penis but identify as being a girl (or have a vulva but identify as being a boy). So, we don't say that all boys have a penis. We say that most boys have a penis, but some don't. And the same for vulvas. If you explain this in a matter of fact way, your child won't find this confusing. If they can accept that it is okay to have different color skin or eye colors, then they will accept that not all boys have penises. You can learn more about how to talk to your child about gender and sex here – https://sexedrescue.com/how-to-explain-transgender-to-a-child/

Because you are a female. Penises are what males usually have.

Because you are a male. Vulvas are what females usually have.

Why don't I have breasts?

Because only adults have breasts. We all have nipples, though.

Why do you have hair down there?

Because I'm an adult.

EXTRA INFO: You will have hair down there someday too.

Why do you have blood coming out of your vagina?

Kids associate blood with pain or something scary. So, your child may need reassurance that there is nothing wrong with you.

This is something that female bodies do each month. There is nothing wrong with me.

EXTRA INFO: That is called a period. It happens to all females when they grow up.

 You can access my FREE sex education course for parents at https://sexedrescue.com/back-to-basics/

4 YEAR OLDS

Baby making

Where do babies come from?

They don't want to know about sex. They just want to know where they were before they were born.

Babies come from inside the mommy, from the uterus.

EXTRA INFO: The uterus is like a balloon, and it can stretch and get bigger and bigger. It will get very big as the baby grows inside. It will shrink back down to its normal size once the baby is born.

Where does the baby grow?

The baby grows inside a special bag that is near the mommy's belly.

EXTRA INFO: The proper name for this place is the uterus.

How does the baby get out?

The baby will come out through the vagina (or between the legs) or through a special cut in the mother's belly.

EXTRA INFO: The vagina will stretch open (like a balloon) and let the baby out.

Does having a baby hurt?

It can hurt, but there are doctors and midwives there, and they can help to stop it from hurting too much.

How are babies made?

To make a baby, you need a part from a male and a part from a female.

OR

To make a baby, you need sperm from a male and an egg from a female.

EXTRA INFO: The two parts join together and begin to grow into a baby.

How does the baby get into the uterus?

The male puts their sperm inside the female, where it then joins with the egg to make a baby.

How does the sperm get into the egg?

The sperm leave the penis and go into the vagina. The egg and sperm join together and grow into a baby.

EXTRA INFO: The male puts their penis into the female's vagina OR the female lets the male put their penis into their vagina.

How was I made?

Babies can be made in lots of different ways: sexual intercourse, sperm and/or egg donation, assisted reproductive technology, surrogacy, adoption. You can find children's books that will help with explaining the way your child was made in this list - http://booksfordonoroffspring.blogspot.com/

Natural conception (penis in vagina sex)

Babies can be made in lots of different ways, but we made you all by ourselves by having sex (or sexual intercourse).

EXTRA INFO: Babies can be made in lots of different ways, and some parents need help to make their baby.

Sperm and/or egg donation

Babies can be made in lots of different ways, but we needed some help to make you. Someone gave us some sperm/eggs, and some doctors helped us to make you.

Assisted Reproductive Technology

Babies can be made in lots of different ways, but we needed some help to make you. A doctor helped to get the sperm and egg to meet, and then they put you in my uterus, which is where you grew.

Surrogacy

Babies can be made in lots of different ways, but we needed some help to make you. We didn't have a uterus, so we found a nice person who grew you inside them until you were born. A doctor helped to get the sperm and egg to meet, and then put you inside a female, which is where you grew.

Adoption

The sperm and egg that made you didn't come from us. You were already growing in the uterus of the person who gave birth to you.

Can we have a new baby?

Keep your answer simple. They don't need to know why!

Yes   No   Maybe

Can I make a baby?

No, not yet. Only adults can have babies.

Can a male/man have a baby?

Technically, some males can have a baby i.e. a transgender man may still have a uterus, which means they can become pregnant. At this age, though, just keep it simple!

You need a uterus to grow a baby.

EXTRA INFO: If a transman has a uterus, they could grow a baby.

Relationships

Regardless of your beliefs, children should be aware that sometimes we grow up and are attracted to the same sex and not the opposite sex. One in ten children grow up being attracted to the same sex, which means your child has a one in ten chance of being same-sex attracted.

All children need to know that sexual orientation is not a choice, all people deserve respect regardless of their sexual orientation, and who we are attracted to, whether it be females or males, is only a small part of who we are.

Try to discuss this topic with care and sensitivity, regardless of your beliefs. Sexual attraction is not a choice. If your child ends up being attracted to the same sex, how will they feel about it and will they feel safe talking to you about it?

If you explain this in a matter of fact way, your child won't find this confusing, especially if they are seeing same-sex couples within your community.

Why are those 2 men (or women) kissing?

Because they like each other, just like me and your mom/dad like each other.

Why does my friend have two mommies (or daddies)?

People fall in love. Some people fall in love with people who are of the same sex, and some don't.

Who will I fall in love with?

I don't know. You will have to wait and see what happens when you are an adult.

EXTRA INFO: It could be a male (or boy), or it could be a female (or girl). When the time is right, you will know the right person for you.

Bodies

Learn more about teaching your child the names of their genitals in this article – https://sexedrescue.com/naming-private-parts/. You can find child-friendly diagrams to show your child here - https://sexedrescue.com/products/. And you can find books for talking to your child about their body here - https://sexedrescue.com/childrens-books-about-private-parts/.

What's this part called?

Just name the body part in your normal everyday voice. You can start off with penis and scrotum (or testicles) or vulva and vagina. You can add in the other parts (foreskin, urethra, clitoris) if you want or name then when your child asks or as they get older. Try to keep it simple!

That's called a ...

Why does my penis go hard? (erection)

> You can let them know that erections have a sexual purpose when they are a bit older and curious about sexual intercourse. At the moment, though, it is just an amazing thing that their body can do.

That is what penises can do.

EXTRA INFO: It is called an erection.

EXTRA INFO: Why? It just shows that your penis is working properly.

Why does my vulva/vagina tickle?

> Don't forget to remind your child that masturbation is a private activity that should happen in a private place. It can take a while for them to understand this concept. You can learn more about how to talk in this article - https://sexedrescue.com/child-masturbation/

Sometimes it does tickle (or feel nice) when you touch yourself.

EXTRA INFO: That is just something that our bodies do, and it means that your body is working properly.

Do I have a uterus and eggs?

> If your child asks why some people don't, just explain that most female bodies do, but that some female bodies don't. It is just something that happens when their body is being made inside their mommy's uterus.

Most females have a uterus and eggs.

EXTRA INFO: But some don't.

Do I have sperm?

Technically, not all males make sperm. They might have something wrong with the part of their body that makes sperm. Or they may be a transwoman (meaning they may still have male parts that make sperm).

Most males will make sperm when they are an adult.

Why don't I have a penis (or vulva)?

Today, we are aware that gender (boy or girl) does not always match your sex (male or female). Some children are intersex (their genitals do not look male or female) or they may have a penis but identify as being a girl (or have a vulva but identify as being a boy). So, we don't say that all boys have a penis. We say that most boys have a penis, but some don't. And the same for vulvas. If you explain this in a matter of fact way, your child won't find this confusing. If they can accept that it is okay to have different color skin or eye colors, then they will accept that not all boys have penises. You can learn more about how to talk to your child about gender and sex here — https://sexedrescue.com/how-to-explain-transgender-to-a-child/

Because you are a female. Penises are what males usually have.

Because you are a male. Vulvas are what females usually have.

Why don't I have breasts?

Because only adults have breasts. We all have nipples, though.

Why do you have hair down there?

Because I'm an adult, and all adults grow hair down there.

EXTRA INFO: I also have hair under my arms, on my legs…

Why do you have blood coming out of your vagina?

Kids associate blood with pain or something scary. So, your child may need reassurance that there is nothing wrong with you.

This is something that my body does each month when there is no baby growing inside of me. There is nothing wrong with me.

EXTRA INFO: That is called my period. It happens to all adult females.

What is the belly button for?

The belly button is where the baby was connected to its mommy when it was growing inside them.

EXTRA INFO: The belly button (umbilicus) is where the tube was that connects the baby to the mother. It feeds the baby so that it can keep on growing. When the baby is born, the tube is cut because the baby can now drink milk instead.

Why do some people stand to pee, but others have to sit?

People with a penis can aim where their pee will go, just like you can with a garden hose. People with a vulva have a shorter pee tube that stops at their vulva. Which means they can't aim as well, so they need to sit down.

You can access my FREE sex education course for parents at https://sexedrescue.com/back-to-basics/

5 YEAR OLDS

Babies (and how they are made)

Some kids like to share this amazing information with their friends. So, it is a good idea to ask them not to. Try saying: 'Some parents like to talk to their own kids about where babies come from.'

Where do babies come from?

Babies come from inside the mommy, from the uterus.

EXTRA INFO: The uterus is like a balloon, and it can stretch and get bigger and bigger. It will get very big as the baby grows inside. It will shrink back down to its normal size once the baby is born.

How does the baby get out?

The baby will come out through the vagina (or between the legs) or through a special cut in the mother's belly.

EXTRA INFO: The vagina will stretch open (like a balloon) and let the baby out.

Does having a baby hurt?

It can hurt, but there are doctors and midwives there, and they can help to stop it from hurting too much.

How are babies made?

To make a baby, you need a part from a male and a part from a female.

OR

To make a baby, you need sperm from a male and an egg from a female.

EXTRA INFO: The two parts join together and begin to grow into a baby.

How does the baby get into the uterus?

The male puts their sperm inside the female. It is inside the female that the sperm and egg join and make a baby.

How does the sperm get to the egg?

The sperm leave the male's penis and go into the female's vagina. The egg and sperm join together and grow into a baby.

EXTRA INFO: The male puts their penis into the female's vagina OR the female lets the male put their penis into their vagina.

How do two mommies make a baby?

A male will give one of the mommies some sperm, which will join with their egg and make a baby.

EXTRA INFO: The mommy might put the sperm into their vagina themself, or a special doctor might do this for them.

How do two daddies make a baby?

They will need to find a female who can grow a baby for them. They might use the egg from that female or another egg that someone has given them to use.

What other ways can a baby be made?

Refer to page 50 for explanations of the different ways babies can be made.

Sometimes the egg and sperm just can't get together. When this happens, the male and female need to see special doctors who collect their egg and sperm. The doctor will help the egg and sperm to join together and will then put it back inside the uterus, where it might grow into a baby.

Can I watch you make a baby?

No, you can't. That is a private thing.

Can we have a new baby?

Keep your answer simple. They don't need to know why!

Yes   No   Maybe

Can I make a baby?

No, not yet. Only adults can have babies.

Can a male/man have a baby?

Technically, some males can have a baby i.e. a transgender man may still have a uterus, which means they can become pregnant. At this age, though, just keep it simple!

You need a uterus to grow a baby.

EXTRA INFO: If a transman has a uterus, they could grow a baby.

Relationships

Regardless of your beliefs, children should be aware that sometimes we grow up and are attracted to the same sex and not the opposite sex. One in ten children grow up being attracted to the same sex, which means your child has a one in ten chance of being same-sex attracted.

All children need to know that sexual orientation is not a choice, all people deserve respect regardless of their sexual orientation, and who we are attracted to, whether it be females or males, is only a small part of who we are.

Try to discuss this topic with care and sensitivity, regardless of your beliefs. Sexual attraction is not a choice. If your child ends up being attracted to the same sex, how will they feel about it and will they feel safe talking to you about it?

If you explain this in a matter of fact way, your child won't find this confusing, especially if they are seeing same-sex couples within your community.

Why are those 2 men (or women) kissing?

Because they like each other, just like me and your mom/dad like each other.

Why does my friend have two mommies (or daddies)?

People fall in love. Some people fall in love with people who are of the same sex, some don't.

What does gay mean?

Gay can mean when a male loves a male or a female loves a female.

EXTRA INFO: Another word for it is homosexual.

Who will I fall in love with?

I don't know. You will have to wait and see what happens when you are a grownup.

EXTRA INFO: It could be a male (or boy), or it could be a female (or girl). When the time is right, you will know the right person for you.

Can I marry you when I am grown up?

Wanting to marry you (or their siblings) is an age-appropriate stage they will outgrow.

No, kids can't marry their mommies or daddies. But don't worry, I will still be your mommy/daddy when you are grown up.

EXTRA INFO: It is against the law for children to marry someone in their family. These are the rules.

Can I marry my sister/brother?

No, kids can't marry their brothers or sisters.

EXTRA INFO: It is against the law for children to marry someone in their family. These are the rules.

Can I marry my friend (opposite sex)?

It very age-appropriate to want to marry their friends. They are seeing couple relationships everywhere and are just copying it.

One day, when you are both all grown up, you can marry your friend. That's up to you!

EXTRA INFO: You don't get married until you are an adult.

Can I marry my friend (same sex)?

Some kids will want to marry their friend who may be the same sex as them. It doesn't mean that your child will be same-sex attracted. They are seeing couple relationships everywhere and are just copying it. So sometimes it is just easier to be neutral with your comments, e.g. 'Yes, dear,' and not make a fuss about it.

One day, when you are both all grown up, you can marry your friend.

EXTRA INFO: You don't get married until you are an adult.

Can I have a boy/girlfriend (special friend)?

Don't get too alarmed if your child starts talking about having a special friend. They see relationships everywhere and just want to copy. The best approach is to be neutral with your comments, i.e. don't make a big fuss about them being too young. It is an age-appropriate phase that they will usually outgrow! Some kids, though, don't outgrow it and may have one 'special friend' for a long time. These relationships are usually very platonic and they aren't usually too upset when they are ended. Try asking a few questions first, i.e. find out why so that you can gauge where they got this idea from.

So, how do you respond? You could just ignore it and go, 'Yes, dear.' Or you could say that that there is no rush for boy/girlfriends, and that is the sort of thing that they will do when they are grown up or a bit older. At the end of the day, do what feels right for you. The important thing is to not make a big deal about it, as it is just a stage that they will usually outgrow.

Yes   No   You can when you are older

Bodies

Learn more about teaching your child the names of their genitals in this article — https://sexedrescue.com/naming-private-parts/. You can find child-friendly diagrams to show your child here - https://sexedrescue.com/products/. And you can find books for talking to your child about their body here - https://sexedrescue.com/childrens-books-about-private-parts/.

What's this part called?

Just name the body part in your normal everyday voice. You can start off with penis and scrotum (or testicles) or vulva and vagina. You can add in the other parts (foreskin, urethra, clitoris) if you want or name then when your child asks or as they get older. Try to keep it simple!

That's called a ...

Why does my penis go hard? (erection)

You can let them know that erections have a sexual purpose when they are a bit older and curious about sexual intercourse. At the moment, though, it is just an amazing thing that their body can do.

That is what penises can do.

EXTRA INFO: It is called an erection.

EXTRA INFO: Why? It just shows that your penis is working properly

Why does my vulva/vagina tickle?

Don't forget to remind your child that masturbation is a private activity that should happen in a private place. It can take a while for them to understand this concept. You can learn more about child masturbation in this article - https://sexedrescue.com/child-masturbation/

Sometimes it does tickle (or feel nice) when you touch yourself.

EXTRA INFO: That is just something that our bodies do, and it means that your body is working properly.

Do I have a uterus and eggs?

If your child asks why some people don't, just explain that most female bodies do, but that some female bodies don't. It is just something that happens when their body is being made inside their mommy's uterus.

Only female bodies have a uterus and eggs.

Do I have sperm?

Technically, not all males make sperm. They might have something wrong with the part of their body that makes sperm. Or they may be a transwoman (meaning they may still have male parts which make sperm).

Most males will make sperm when they are an adult.

No. Only grown up male bodies make sperm.

OR

No. Most males will make sperm when they are an adult, but some don't.

Why don't I have a penis (or vulva)?

Today, we are aware that gender (boy or girl) does not always match your sex (male or female). Some children are intersex (their genitals do not look male or female) or they may have a penis but identify as being a girl (or have a vulva but identify as being a boy). So, we don't say that all boys have a penis. We say that most boys have a penis, but some don't. And the same for vulvas. If you explain this in a matter of fact way, your child won't find this confusing. If they can accept that it is okay to have different color skin or eye colors, then they will accept that not all boys have penises. You can learn more about how to talk to your child about gender and sex here — https://sexedrescue.com/how-to-explain-transgender-to-a-child/

Because you are a female. Penises are what males usually have.

Because you are a male. Vulvas are what females usually have.

Why don't I have breasts?

Because only adults have breasts. We all have nipples, though.

Why do you have hair down there?

Because I'm an adult, and all adults grow hair down there.

EXTRA INFO: I also have hair under my arms, on my legs…

Why do you have blood coming out of your vagina?

Kids associate blood with pain or something scary. So, your child may need reassurance that there is nothing wrong with you.

That is my period. It doesn't hurt and just looks like blood. Most women have their period every month.

EXTRA INFO: Every month my body gets ready to have a baby. My uterus grows a thin layer of blood and special tissue that make a soft bed for a baby to grow on. If I'm not pregnant, my body throws the bed as way, as it isn't needed. It comes out as blood through my vagina. This is called having a period.

What is the belly button for?

The belly button is where the baby was connected to its mommy when it was growing inside them.

EXTRA INFO: The belly button (umbilicus) is where the tube was that connects the baby to the mother. It feeds the baby so that it can keep on growing. When the baby is born, the tube is cut because the baby can now drink milk instead.

Why do some people stand to pee, but others have to sit?

People with a penis can aim where their pee will go, just like you can with a garden hose. People with a vulva have a shorter pee tube that stops at their vulva. Which means they can't aim as well, so they need to sit down.

 You can access my FREE sex education course for parents at https://sexedrescue.com/back-to-basics/

6 YEAR OLDS

Babies (and how they are made)

Some kids like to share this amazing information with their friends. So, it is a good idea to ask them not to. Try saying: 'Some parents like to talk to their own kids about where babies come from.'

How are babies made?

To make a baby, you need sperm from a male and an egg from a female. The **2** parts join together and turn into a baby.

Where does the baby grow?

The baby grows inside a special bag that is near the mother's stomach.

EXTRA INFO: The proper name for this place is the uterus.

How does the baby get out?

The baby will come out through the vagina (or between the legs) OR through a special cut in my tummy. The vagina will stretch open (like a balloon) and let the baby out.

Does having a baby hurt?

It can hurt, but there are doctors and midwives there, and they can help to stop it from hurting too much.

How does the baby get into the uterus?

The male puts their sperm inside the female. It is inside the female that the sperm and egg join and make a baby.

How does the sperm get to the egg?

The sperm leave the penis and go into the vagina. The egg and sperm join together and grow into a baby.

EXTRA INFO: The male puts their penis into the female's vagina OR the female lets the male put their penis into their vagina.

How do the penis and vagina meet?

Kids sometimes get confused and think that the male removes their penis to do this.

The male places their penis into the vagina. OR the female lets the male place their penis into the vagina.

EXTRA INFO: The male and female have sex (sexual intercourse). They hold each other close, then the penis goes hard and is put into the vagina. Sex is something that is just for adults.

What other ways can a baby be made?

Refer to page 50 for explanations of the different ways babies can be made.

Sometimes the egg and sperm just can't get together. When this happens, the male and female need to see special doctors who collect their egg and sperm. The doctor will help the egg and sperm to join together and will then put it back inside the uterus, where it might grow into a baby.

How do two females make a baby?

A male will give one of the females some sperm, which will join with the egg and make a baby.

EXTRA INFO: The female might put the sperm into their vagina themself, or a special doctor might do this for them.

How do two males make a baby?

They will need to find a female who can grow a baby for them. They might use the egg from that person or another egg that someone has given them to use.

Can I watch you make a baby?

No, you can't. That is a private thing.

Can we have a new baby?

Keep your answer simple. They don't need to know why!

Yes   No   Maybe

Can I Make a baby?

No, not yet. Only adults can have babies.

EXTRA INFO: You won't be able to make a baby until after puberty.

Can a male/man have a baby?

Technically, some men can have a baby, i.e. a transgender male may still have a uterus, which means they can become pregnant.

You need a uterus to grow a baby, so it is usually females (or women) that have babies.

EXTRA INFO: Sometimes a female doesn't feel like a girl on the inside. When they are grown up, they might dress and act like a man, even though they have a vagina. Or they might have a special operation that turns them into a male on the outside. If they leave the uterus (baby bag) in, it means that they could one day have a baby.

Sexual activities (including intercourse)

Some kids like to share this amazing information with their friends. So, it is a good idea to ask them not to. Try saying: 'Some parents like to talk to their own kids about sexual intercourse.'

Your child will hear about sex at the playground, from their friends and through the media. This means that you have to be prepared for questions about sexual activities that are not age-appropriate, like bestiality (having sex with animals). Answering their questions will satisfy their curiosity and allow them to move on to something else, like, 'What's for dinner?' If you don't satisfy their curiosity, they may just go looking for an answer elsewhere, e.g. their friends or the internet.

If your child starts to ask questions about the different types of sexual behavior, it is usually a good idea to find out why they are asking the question. You could very casually say, 'Why are you asking that?' or, 'Where did you hear that word?'

When talking to kids about sex, you can add a value statement about the situations in which you believe sex should happen, e.g. 'In our family, we believe that you shouldn't have sex until...' (you are married, in a loving and committed relationship, are 16, or whatever it is that you believe in).

What is sex?

At first, kids are only curious about sex because they want to know how babies are made or they have heard whispers and giggles about this thing called sex. So, when we first start talking about sex, we can just talk about baby-making sex, i.e. sexual intercourse. Later on, we start adding in that there is a bit more to sex, like hugging, kissing, etc. And that adults also have sex for other reasons as well. And we always remind kids that sex is something that adults do and that it is not for kids.

Sex is something that adults do when they want to make a baby.

EXTRA INFO: Sex can be lots of different things. Sex or sexual intercourse is when the male's penis gets stiff, and is then put into the female's vagina (or the female lets the male place their penis into the vagina). This is something that is just for adults.

What happens when you have sex?

There are lots of different ways to have sex. The main way that adults have sex to make a baby is when the penis goes into the vagina. They also do other things like hug, kiss, and touch each other's bodies in a nice way.

EXTRA INFO: Sex is something that most people do when they are grown up.

Will I have sex one day?

Yes, you probably will have sex one day, but it won't be until you are an adult.

What does sexy mean?

Sexy is a word that adults might use to describe someone that they think is attractive. It is a word that adults use.

You can add a value statement if you don't want your child to use this word, e.g. 'Sexy is not a word that we use in our family.'

What is oral sex?

Your child may hear other kids talking about oral sex and may be curious as to what it means. Remember to ask them why they are asking, just in case there is another reason for their question.

Oral sex is when people put their mouths on someone else's penis or vulva. This is something that is just for grown-ups.

What is anal sex?

Your child may hear other kids talking about anal sex and may be curious as to what it means. Remember to ask them why they are asking, just in case there is another reason for their question.

Anal sex is when the penis goes into the anus (or bottom). This is something that is just for adults.

What is a condom?

Your child may hear other kids talking about condoms and may be curious as to what it means. Or they may find one on the ground at the park. Remember to ask them why they are asking, just in case there is another reason for their question.

A condom is something that people use when they don't want to have babies.

EXTRA INFO: It is like a long skinny balloon, and it covers the penis.

Masturbation

You will need to talk with your child about what your family values and beliefs are on masturbation. Try to talk about this in a way that will not leave your child feeling shame and guilt. Kids just see it as a part of their body that feels good when you touch it. We now see it as a normal sexual behaviour that is not harmful.

You can learn more about how to talk in this article - https://sexedrescue.com/child-masturbation/

Don't forget to remind your child that this is a private activity that should happen in a private place. It can take a while for them to understand this concept of private.

What is masturbation?

Masturbation is when you touch your penis or clitoris/vulva in a nice way and it feels nice.

Why does my vulva/vagina/penis tickle?

Sometimes it does tickle (or feel nice) when you touch yourself.

EXTRA INFO: That is just something that our bodies do, and it means that your body is working properly.

Relationships

Regardless of your beliefs, children should be aware that sometimes we grow up and are attracted to the same sex and not the opposite sex. One in ten children grow up being attracted to the same sex, which means your child has a one in ten chance of being same-sex attracted.

All children need to know that sexual orientation is not a choice, all people deserve respect regardless of their sexual orientation, and who we are attracted to, whether it be females or males, is only a small part of who we are.

Try to discuss this topic with care and sensitivity, regardless of your beliefs. Sexual attraction is not a choice. If your child ends up being attracted to the same sex, how will they feel about it and will they feel safe talking to you about it?

If you explain this in a matter of fact way, your child won't find this confusing, especially if they are seeing same-sex couples within your community.

Why are those 2 men (or women) kissing?

Because they like each other, just like me and your mom/dad like each other.

Why does my friend have two mommies?

Some people fall in love with people who are of the same sex, and some don't.

What does gay mean?

Gay can mean when a male loves a male or a female loves a female.

EXTRA INFO: Another word for it is homosexual.

Who will I fall in love with?

I don't know. You will have to wait and see what happens when you are a grownup.

EXTRA INFO: It could be a male (or boy), or it could be a female (or girl). When the time is right, you will know the right person for you.

Can I marry you when I am grown up?

Wanting to marry you (or their siblings) is an age-appropriate stage they will outgrow.

No, kids can't marry their mommies or daddies. But don't worry, I will still be your mommy/daddy when you are grown up.

EXTRA INFO: It is against the law for children to marry someone in their family. These are the rules.

Can I marry my sister/brother?

No, kids can't marry their brothers or sisters.

EXTRA INFO: It is against the law for children to marry someone in their family. These are the rules.

Can I marry my friend (opposite sex)?

It very age-appropriate to want to marry their friends. They are seeing couple relationships everywhere and are just copying it.

One day, when you are both all grown up, you can marry your friend. That's up to you!

EXTRA INFO: You don't get married until you are an adult.

Can I marry my friend (same sex)?

Some kids will want to marry their friend who may be the same sex as them. It doesn't mean that your child will be same-sex attracted. They are seeing couple relationships everywhere and are just copying it. So, sometimes it is just easier to be neutral with your comments, e.g. 'Yes, dear,' and not make a fuss about it.

One day, when you are both all grown up, you can marry your friend.

EXTRA INFO: You don't get married until you are an adult.

Can I have a boy/girlfriend (special friend)?

Don't get too alarmed if your child starts talking about having a special friend. They see relationships everywhere and just want to copy. The best approach is to be neutral with your comments, i.e. don't make a big fuss about them being too young. It is an age-appropriate phase that they will usually outgrow! Some kids, though, don't outgrow it and may have one 'special friend' for a long time. These relationships are usually very platonic and they aren't usually too upset when they are ended. Try asking a few questions first, i.e. find out why so that you can gauge where they got this idea from.

So, how do you respond? You could just ignore it and go, 'Yes, dear.' Or you could say that that there is no rush for boy/girlfriends, and that is the sort of thing that they will do when they are grown up or a bit older. At the end of the day, do what feels right for you. The important thing is to not make a big deal about it, as it is just a stage that they will usually outgrow.

Yes   No   You can when you are older

Bodies

Learn more about teaching your child the names of their genitals in this article — https://sexedrescue.com/naming-private-parts/. You can find child-friendly diagrams to show your child here - https://sexedrescue.com/products/. And you can find books for talking to your child about their body here - https://sexedrescue.com/childrens-books-about-private-parts/.

What's this part called?

Just name the body part in your normal everyday voice. You can start off with penis and scrotum (or testicles) or vulva and vagina. You can add in the other parts (foreskin, urethra, clitoris) if you want or name then when your child asks or as they get older. Try to keep it simple!

That's called a ...

Why does my penis go hard? (erection)

You can let them know that erections have a sexual purpose when they are a bit older and curious about sexual intercourse. At the moment, though, it is just an amazing thing that their body can do.

That is what penises can do.

EXTRA INFO: It is called an erection.

EXTRA INFO: Why? It just shows that your penis is working properly

Why is my friend's penis different?

Some penises are circumcised. This means that the skin on the end of their penis has been cut off. This means that the penis will look a little different at the end.

EXTRA INFO: Circumcision can happen for religious or cultural reasons or because the foreskin can't stretch enough to be pushed back.

Do I have a uterus and eggs?

If your child asks why some people don't, just explain that most female bodies do, but that some female bodies don't. It is just something that happens when their body is being made inside their mommy's uterus.

Only female bodies have a uterus and eggs

EXTRA INFO: Some female bodies don't have them. Why? For some reason, their body was just made differently.

Do I have sperm?

Technically, not all males make sperm. They might have something wrong with the part of their body that makes sperm. Or they may be a transwoman (meaning they may still have male parts that make sperm).

No. Only grown up male bodies make sperm.

OR

No. Most males will make sperm when they are an adult, but some don't.

Why don't I have a penis (or vulva)?

Today, we are aware that gender (boy or girl) does not always match your sex (male or female). Some children are intersex (their genitals do not look male or female) or they may have a penis but identify as being a girl (or have a vulva but identify as being a boy). So, we don't say that all boys have a penis. We say that most boys have a penis, but some don't. And the same for vulvas. If you explain this in a matter of fact way, your child won't find this confusing. If they can accept that it is okay to have different color skin or eye colors, then they will accept that not all boys have penises. You can learn more about how to talk to your child about gender and sex here — https://sexedrescue.com/how-to-explain-transgender-to-a-child/

Because you are a female. Penises are what males usually have.

Because you are a male. Vulvas are what females usually have.

Why don't I have breasts?

Because only adults have breasts. We all have nipples, though.

Why do you have hair down there?

Because I'm an adult, and all adults grow hair down there.

EXTRA INFO: I also have hair under my arms, on my legs…

Why do you have blood coming out of your vagina?

Kids associate blood with pain or something scary. So, your child may need reassurance that there is nothing wrong with you.

That is my period. It doesn't hurt and just looks like blood. Most women have their period every month.

EXTRA INFO: Every month, my body gets ready to have a baby. My uterus grows a thin layer of blood and special tissue that makes a soft bed for a baby to grow on. If I'm not pregnant, my body throws the bed as way, as it isn't needed. It comes out as blood through my vagina. This is called having a period.

What is the belly button for?

The belly button is where the baby was connected to its mommy when it was growing inside them.

EXTRA INFO: The belly button (umbilicus) is where the tube was that connects the baby to the mother. It feeds the baby so that it can keep on growing. When the baby is born, the tube is cut because the baby can now drink milk instead.

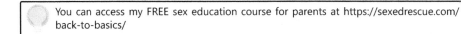 You can access my FREE sex education course for parents at https://sexedrescue.com/back-to-basics/

7 YEAR OLDS

Babies (and how they are made)

Some kids like to share this amazing information with their friends. So, it is a good idea to ask them not to. Try saying: 'Some parents like to talk to their own kids about where babies come from.'

Try to get into the habit of explaining what you think or believe when talking about love, sex and relationships. This is your opportunity to guide your child as they grow up, and to help them make healthy decisions around love, sex and relationships.

How are babies made?

To make a baby, you need sperm from a male and an egg from a female. The **2** parts join together and turn into a baby.

Where does the baby grow?

The baby grows inside a special bag that is near the mother's stomach.

EXTRA INFO: The proper name for this place is the uterus.

How does the baby get out?

The baby will come out through the vagina (or between the legs) OR through a special cut in my tummy.

EXTRA INFO: The vagina will stretch open (like a balloon) and let the baby out.

Does having a baby hurt?

It can hurt, but there are doctors and midwives there, and they can help to stop it from hurting too much.

How does the baby get into the uterus?

The male has to put their sperm inside the female. It is inside the female that the two parts join and make a baby.

How does the sperm get to the egg?

If your child was made differently, you could explain the way that they were made. Refer to page 50 for an explanation.

The sperm leave the penis and go into the vagina. The egg and sperm join together and grow into a baby.

EXTRA INFO: The male puts their penis into the female's vagina OR the female lets the male put their penis into their vagina.

How do the penis and vagina meet?

Kids sometimes get confused and think that the male removes their penis to do this.

The male puts their penis into the vagina OR the female lets the male put their penis into their vagina.

EXTRA INFO: The male and female have sex (sexual intercourse). They hold each other close, then the penis goes hard and is put into the vagina (or the female lets the male place their penis in the vagina). Sperm comes out of the penis into the vagina. The sperm then travels up inside the uterus, looking for an egg to fertilize (or turn into a baby). A baby may (or may not) happen. Sex is something that is just for adults.

What other ways can a baby be made?

Refer to page 50 for explanations of the different ways babies can be made.

Sometimes the egg and sperm just can't get together. When this happens, the male and female need to see special doctors who collect their egg and sperm. The doctor will help the egg and sperm to join together and will then put it back inside the uterus, where it might grow into a baby.

How do two females make a baby?

A male will give one of the females some sperm, which will join with the egg and make a baby.

EXTRA INFO: The female might put the sperm into their vagina themself, or a special doctor might do this for them.

How do two males make a baby?

They will need to find a female who can grow a baby for them. They might use the egg from that person or another egg that someone has given them to use.

How is the egg made?

Females are born with their eggs already inside them.

EXTRA INFO: Eggs are found inside the ovaries.

How does the sperm find the egg?

The sperm are like tadpoles. They swim through the vagina and go up into the uterus, looking for an egg to fertilize.

How does the sperm fertilize the egg?

When the sperm find the egg, one of them will push and wiggle itself inside the egg.

EXTRA INFO: The egg closes up the hole, and then the egg and sperm become one cell – the beginning cell of a baby.

How is the egg made into a baby?

Once the sperm joins with the egg, it begins to divide into even more cells. This creates something called DNA, which is like a set of instructions on how the baby should grow.

How long does it take to make a baby?

This answer is based on how long it can take for the male to ejaculate with vaginal penetration.

Not very long. It can happen within a couple of minutes.

How long does it take for the sperm to find the egg?

Anywhere from half an hour to 5 days.

Do you have to have sex every time you want a baby?

Yes, usually you do.

EXTRA INFO: Sometimes you don't need to have sex to make a baby. Sometimes the people need help to get the egg and sperm together. This means that they need to get some special doctors to help the egg and sperm to join together to make a baby. This can happen for a lot of different medical reasons.

How many times do you need to have sex to make a baby?

You only need to have sex once to make a baby, but sometimes it takes more than one time to make a baby.

Can I have a baby?

No, not yet. Only adults can have babies.

How old do you have to be to have a baby?

Males need to be making sperm before they can help to make a baby. So that could be anytime from the age of **13** or **14**.

Females need to be having their periods before they can become pregnant. So that could be anytime from the age of **10-11**.

You can also add a value statement about when you feel they should be having babies, e.g. 'In our family, we believe that you shouldn't have sex until...' (you are married, in a loving and committed relationship, are 16 or whatever it is that you believe in).

Can a male/man have a baby?

Technically, some men can have a baby, i.e. a transgender male may still have a uterus, which means they can become pregnant.

You need a uterus to grow a baby, so it is usually females (or women) that have babies.

EXTRA INFO: Sometimes a female doesn't feel like a girl on the inside. When they are grown up, they might dress and act like a man, even though they have a vagina. Or they might have a special operation that turns them into a male on the outside. If they leave the uterus (baby bag) in, it means that they could one day have a baby.

Sexual activities (including intercourse)

Some kids like to share this amazing information with their friends. So, it is a good idea to ask them not to. Try saying: 'Some parents like to talk to their own kids about sexual intercourse.'

Your child will hear about sex at the playground, from their friends and through the media. This means that you have to be prepared for questions about sexual activities that are not age-appropriate, like bestiality (having sex with animals). Answering their questions will satisfy their curiosity and allow them to move on to something else, like, 'What's for dinner?' If you don't satisfy their curiosity, they may just go looking for an answer elsewhere, e.g. their friends or the internet.

If your child starts to ask questions about the different types of sexual behavior, it is usually a good idea to find out why they are asking the question. You could very casually say, 'Why are you asking that?' or, 'Where did you hear that word?'

When talking to kids about sex, you can add a value statement about the situations in which you believe sex should happen, e.g. 'In our family, we believe that you shouldn't have sex until...' (you are married, in a loving and committed relationship, are 16, or whatever it is that you believe in).

What is sex?

At first, kids are only curious about sex because they want to know how babies are made or they have heard whispers and giggles about this thing called sex. So, when we first start talking about sex (sexual intercourse), we can just talk about baby-making sex, i.e. sexual intercourse. Later on, we start adding in that there is a bit more to sex like hugging, kissing, etc. And that adults also have sex for other reasons as well. And we always remind kids that sex is something that adults do and that it is not for kids.

Sex is something that adults can do when they want to make a baby.

EXTRA INFO: Sex can be lots of different things. Sex or sexual intercourse is when the penis gets stiff, and they then put it into the vagina (or the female lets the male put their penis into the vagina). They also do other things like hug,

85

kiss, and touch each other's bodies in a nice way. This is something that is just for adults.

What happens when you have sex?

Eventually your child will realize that adults don't just have sex to make babies. So, you can also start talking about how adults often kiss, hug, touch and engage in other sexual behaviors with one another to show caring for each other and to feel good.

There are lots of different ways to have sex. The main way that adults have sex to make a baby is when the penis goes into the vagina. They also do other things like hug, kiss, and touch each other's bodies in a nice way.

EXTRA INFO: Sex is something that most people do when they are grown up.

How do two females have sex?

You don't need to go into great detail here. Keep it simple!

There is more to sex than penises and vaginas. It is also about kissing, hugging, and touching each other's genitals. Gay (or lesbian) females can do all of this except for putting a penis in a vagina.

How do two males have sex?

You don't need to go into great detail here. Keep it simple!

There is more to sex than penises and vaginas. It is also about kissing, hugging, and touching each other's genitals. Gay males can do all of this except for putting a penis in a vagina.

Will I have sex one day?

Yes, you probably will have sex one day, but it won't be until you are an adult.

Why do people have sex?

Adults have sex for lots of different reasons. To make babies, to show their love for each other, and even for fun.

EXTRA INFO: Parents have sex and enjoy it. It is something that parents do.

Where do adults have sex?

Usually somewhere private, like in their bedroom.

EXTRA INFO: Sex is a private activity.

Do you have to lie down to have sex?

If you want to, you can. There are lots of different ways that adults can position their bodies to have sexual intercourse.

Do you have to be married to have sex?

The answer to this question depends on your personal beliefs.

Yes, in our family/church, we believe that you need to be married to have sex.

OR

No, in our family we don't believe that you need to be married first. But we believe that you need to be an adult and in a loving and committed relationship first (or say what you believe in).

EXTRA INFO: But, physically, your grownup body is capable of having sex whether you are married or not.

Does it hurt to have sex?

> Sometimes sex does hurt, but kids don't need to know about sexual pain yet.

No, sex doesn't hurt. Sex can feel really good.

EXTRA INFO: Your body is designed so that it won't hurt.

How old do you have to be to have sex?

> This answer depends on the law in the country and/or state that you live in. If you are unsure, just google 'legal age for sexual consent in (your state or country).'

The law says that you have to be (the legal age where you live). But in our family, we think that you shouldn't have sex until...' (you are married, in a loving and committed relationship, or whatever it is that you believe in).

What does sexy mean?

Sexy is a word that adults might use to describe someone that they think is attractive. It is a word that adults use.

You can add a value statement if you don't want your child to use this word, e.g. 'Sexy is not a word that we use in our family.'

What is oral sex?

> Your child may hear other kids talking about oral sex and may be curious as to what it means. Remember to ask them why they are asking, just in case there is another reason for their question.

Oral sex is when people put their mouths on someone else's penis or vulva. This is something that is just for adults.

What is anal sex?

Your child may hear other kids talking about anal sex and may be curious as to what it means. Remember to ask them why they are asking, just in case there is another reason for their question.

Anal sex is when the penis goes into the anus (or bottom). This is something that is just for adults.

What is a condom?

A condom is something that people use when they don't want to have babies.

EXTRA INFO: It is like a long, skinny balloon, and it covers the penis.

Masturbation

You will need to talk with your child about what your family values and beliefs are on masturbation. Try to talk about this in a way that will not leave your child feeling shame and guilt. Kids just see it as a part of their body that feels good when you touch it. We now see it as a normal sexual behaviour that is not harmful. You can learn more about how to talk in this article - https://sexedrescue.com/child-masturbation/

Don't forget to remind your child that this is a private activity that should happen in a private place.

What is masturbation?

Masturbation is when you touch your penis or clitoris/vulva in a nice way and it feels nice.

Why does my vulva/vagina tickle?

Remind your child that this is a private activity that should happen in a private place. It can take a while for them to understand this concept of private.

Sometimes it does tickle (or feel nice) when you touch yourself.

EXTRA INFO: That is just something that our bodies do, and it means that your body is working properly.

Why does it feel nice when I touch my penis/vulva/clitoris?

Sometimes it does feel nice when you touch yourself down there. That is just something that our bodies do and it means that your body is working properly.

EXTRA INFO: It feels nice because of your clitoris. The clitoris can feel nice when it is touched.

Love and attraction

Regardless of your beliefs, children should be aware that sometimes we grow up and are attracted to the same sex and not the opposite sex. One in ten children grow up being attracted to the same sex, which means your child has a one in ten chance of being same-sex attracted.

All children need to know that sexual orientation is not a choice, all people deserve respect regardless of their sexual orientation, and who we are attracted to, whether it be females or males, is only a small part of who we are.

Try to discuss this topic with care and sensitivity, regardless of your beliefs. Sexual attraction is not a choice. If your child ends up being attracted to the same sex, how will they feel about it and will they feel safe talking to you about it?

If you explain this in a matter of fact way, your child won't find this confusing, especially if they are seeing same-sex couples within your community.

Why are those 2 men (or women) kissing?

Because they like each other, just like me and your mom/dad like each other.

Why does my friend have two mommies?

Some people fall in love with people who are of the same sex, and some don't.

What does gay mean?

Gay can mean when a male loves a male or a female loves a female.

EXTRA INFO: Another word for it is homosexual.

Why are some people gay?

Being attracted to someone of the same sex is just something that happens. You can't stop it from happening. We don't really know why people like someone of the same or opposite sex; it just happens.

Who will I fall in love with?

I don't know. You will have to wait and see what happens when you are an adult.

EXTRA INFO: It could be a male (or boy), or it could be a female (or girl). When the time is right, you will know the right person for you.

Can I have a boy/girlfriend (special friend)?

Don't get too alarmed if your child starts talking about having a special friend. They see relationships everywhere and just want to copy. The best approach is to be neutral with your comments, i.e. don't make a big fuss about them being too young. It is an age-appropriate phase that they will usually outgrow! Some kids, though, don't outgrow it and may have one 'special friend' for a long time. These relationships are usually very platonic and they aren't usually too upset when they are ended. Try asking a few questions first, i.e. find out why so that you can gauge where they got this idea from.

So, how do you respond? You could just ignore it and go, 'Yes, dear.' Or you could say that that there is no rush for boy/girlfriends, and that is the sort of thing that they will do when they are grown up or a bit older. At the end of the day, do what feels right for you. The important thing is to not make a big deal about it, as it is just a stage that they will usually outgrow.

Yes	No	You can when you are older

Bodies

Learn more about teaching your child the names of their genitals in this article — https://sexedrescue.com/naming-private-parts/. You can find child-friendly diagrams to show your child here - https://sexedrescue.com/products/. And you can find books for talking to your child about their body here - https://sexedrescue.com/childrens-books-about-private-parts/.

What's this part called?

Just name the body part in your normal everyday voice. You can start off with penis and scrotum (or testicles) or vulva and vagina. You can add in the other parts (foreskin, urethra, clitoris) if you want or name then when your child asks or as they get older. Try to keep it simple!

That's called a ...

Why does my penis go hard? (erection)

You can let them know that erections have a sexual purpose when they are a bit older and curious about sexual intercourse. At the moment, though, it is just an amazing thing that their body can do.

That is what penises can do. It is called an erection.

EXTRA INFO: Why? It just shows that your penis is working properly.

EXTRA INFO: The penis needs to be hard so that the male can push it inside the vagina during sex.

Why is my friend's penis different?

Some penises are circumcised. This means that the skin on the end of their penis has been cut off. This means that the penis will look a little different at the end.

EXTRA INFO: Circumcision can happen for religious or cultural reasons, or because the foreskin can't stretch enough to be pushed back.

Do I have a uterus and eggs?

If your child asks why some people don't, just explain that most female bodies do, but that some female bodies don't. It is just something that happens when their body is being made inside their mommy's uterus.

Most females have a uterus and eggs, but some don't.

Do I have sperm?

Technically, not all males make sperm. They might have something wrong with the part of their body that makes sperm. Or they may be a transwoman (meaning they may still have male parts that make sperm).

No. Only grown up male bodies make sperm.

OR

No. Most males will make sperm when they are an adult, but some don't.

Why don't I have breasts?

Because only adults have breasts. We all have nipples, though.

Why don't I have a penis (or vulva)?

Today, we are aware that gender (boy or girl) does not always match your sex (male or female). Some children are intersex (their genitals do not look male or female) or they may have a penis but identify as being a girl (or have a vulva but identify as being a boy). So, we don't say that all boys have a penis. We say that most boys have a penis, but some don't. And the same for vulvas. If you explain this in a matter of fact way, your child won't find this confusing. If they can accept that it is okay to have different color skin or eye colors, then they will accept that not all boys have penises. You can learn more about how to talk to your child about gender and sex here — https://sexedrescue.com/how-to-explain-transgender-to-a-child/

Because you are a female. Penises are what males usually have.

Because you are a male. Vulvas are what females usually have.

Why do you have hair down there?

Because I'm an adult, and all adults grow hair down there.

EXTRA INFO: I also have hair under my arms, on my legs…

Why do you have blood coming out of your vagina?

Kids associate blood with pain or something scary. So, your child may need reassurance that there is nothing wrong with you.

That is my period. It doesn't hurt and just looks like blood. Most females have their period every month.

EXTRA INFO: Every month, my body gets ready to have a baby. My uterus grows a thin layer of blood and special tissue that makes a soft bed for a baby to grow on. If I'm not pregnant, my body throws the bed as way, as it isn't needed. It comes out as blood through my vagina. This is called having a period.

 You can access my FREE sex education course for parents at https://sexedrescue.com/back-to-basics/

8 YEAR OLDS

Babies (and how they are made)

Some kids like to share this amazing information with their friends. So, it is a good idea to ask them not to. Try saying: 'Some parents like to talk to their own kids about where babies come from.'

Try to get into the habit of explaining what you think or believe when talking about love, sex and relationships. This is your opportunity to guide your child as they grow up, and to help them make healthy decisions around love, sex and relationships.

How are babies made?

A baby is made (or conceived) when sperm from the male joins with an egg/ovum from the female.

Where does the baby grow?

The baby grows inside a special bag that is near the mother's stomach.

EXTRA INFO: The proper name for this place is the uterus.

How does the baby get out?

The baby will come out through the vagina (or between the legs) OR through a special cut in the tummy. The vagina will stretch open (like a balloon) and let the baby out.

EXTRA INFO: When the baby is ready to be born, the mother goes into labour. This is when the uterus starts to push down around the baby (contract). This helps to push the baby out of the uterus, and into the vagina, which is where it then comes out.

Sometimes the mother needs help getting the baby out. So, the doctor makes a special cut through her stomach and brings the baby out that way. This is called a caesarian or c-section.

Once the baby is born, it can breathe on its own. The umbilical cord is cut, which means that the baby will now be fed with milk. This doesn't hurt the mother or the baby, and the cord falls off in a couple of days, leaving the belly button (navel or umbilicus) behind.

Does having a baby hurt?

It can hurt, but there are doctors and midwives there, and they can help to stop it from hurting too much.

How does the baby get into the uterus?

The male has to put their sperm inside the female. It is inside the female that the two parts join and make a baby.

How does the sperm get to the egg?

If your child was made differently, you could explain the way that they were made. Refer to page 50 for an explanation

The sperm leave the penis and go into the vagina. The egg and sperm join together and grow into a baby.

EXTRA INFO: The male puts their penis into the female's vagina OR the female lets the male put their penis into their vagina.

How do the penis and vagina meet?

Kids sometimes get confused and think that the male removes their penis to do this.

The male puts their penis into the vagina OR the female lets the male put their penis into their vagina.

EXTRA INFO: The male and female have sex (sexual intercourse). They hold each other close, then the male's penis goes hard and is put into the vagina (or the female lets the male place their penis in the vagina). Sperm comes out of the penis into the vagina. The sperm then travels up inside the uterus, looking for an egg to fertilize (or turn into a baby). A baby may (or may not) happen. Sex is something that is just for adults.

What other ways can a baby be made?

Refer to page 50 for explanations of the different ways babies can be made.

Sometimes the egg and sperm just can't get together. When this happens, the male and female need to see special doctors who collect their egg and sperm. The doctor will help the egg and sperm to join together and will then put it back inside the uterus, where it might grow into a baby.

How do two females make a baby?

A male will give one of the females some sperm, which will join with the egg and make a baby.

EXTRA INFO: The female might put the sperm into their vagina themself, or a special doctor might do this for them.

How do two males make a baby?

They will need to find a female who can grow a baby for them. They might use the egg from that person or another egg that someone has given them to use.

How is the egg made?

Females are born with their eggs already inside them.

EXTRA INFO: Eggs are found inside the ovaries.

How does the sperm find the egg?

The sperm are like tadpoles. They swim through the vagina and go up into the uterus, looking for an egg to fertilize.

How does the sperm fertilize the egg?

When the sperm find the egg, one of them will push and wiggle itself inside the egg.

EXTRA INFO: The egg closes up the hole, and then the egg and sperm become one cell – the beginning cell of a baby.

How is the egg made into a baby?

Once the sperm joins with the egg, it begins to divide into even more cells. This creates something called DNA, which is like a set of instructions on how the baby should grow.

How long does it take to make a baby?

This answer is based on how long it can take for the male to ejaculate with vaginal penetration.

Not very long. It can happen within a couple of minutes.

How long does it take for the sperm to find the egg?

Anywhere from half an hour to 5 days.

Do you have to have sex every time you want a baby?

Yes, usually you do.

EXTRA INFO: Sometimes you don't need to have sex to make a baby. Sometimes the people need help to get the egg and sperm together. This means that they need to get some special doctors to help the egg and sperm to join together to make a baby. This can happen for a lot of different medical reasons.

How many times do you need to have sex to make a baby?

You only need to have sex once to make a baby, but sometimes it takes more than one time to make a baby.

How old do you have to be to have a baby?

Males need to be making sperm before they can help to make a baby. So that could be anytime from the age of **13** or **14**.

Females need to be having their periods before they can become pregnant. So that could be anytime from the age of **10-11**.

You can also add a value statement about when you feel they should be having babies, e.g. 'In our family, we believe that you shouldn't have sex until...' (you are married, in a loving and committed relationship, are 16 or whatever it is that you believe in).

Can a male/man have a baby?

Technically, some men can have a baby, i.e. a transgender male may still have a uterus, which means they can become pregnant.

You need a uterus to grow a baby, so it is usually females (or women) that have babies.

EXTRA INFO: Sometimes a female doesn't feel like a girl on the inside. When they are grown up, they might dress and act like a man, even though they have a vagina. Or they might have a special operation that turns them into a male on the outside. If they leave the uterus (baby bag) in, it means that they could one day have a baby.

Sexual activities (including intercourse)

Some kids like to share this amazing information with their friends. So, it is a good idea to ask them not to. Try saying: 'Some parents like to talk to their own kids about sexual intercourse.'

Your child will hear about sex at the playground, from their friends and through the media. This means that you have to be prepared for questions about sexual activities that are not age-appropriate, like bestiality (having sex with animals). Answering their questions will satisfy their curiosity and allow them to move on to something else, like, 'What's for dinner?' If you don't satisfy their curiosity, they may just go looking for an answer elsewhere, e.g. their friends or the internet.

If your child starts to ask questions about the different types of sexual behavior, it is usually a good idea to find out why they are asking the question. You could very casually say, 'Why are you asking that?' or, 'Where did you hear that word?'

When talking to kids about sex, you can add a value statement about the situations in which you believe sex should happen, e.g. 'In our family, we believe that you shouldn't have sex until...' (you are married, in a loving and committed relationship, are 16, or whatever it is that you believe in).

What is sex?

At first, kids are only curious about sex because they want to know how babies are made or they have heard whispers and giggles about this thing called sex. So, when we first start talking about sex (sexual intercourse), we can just talk about baby-making sex, i.e. sexual intercourse. Later on, we start adding in that there is a bit more to sex like hugging, kissing, etc. And that adults also have sex for other reasons as well. And we always remind kids that sex is something that adults do and that it is not for kids.

Sex is something that adults can do when they want to make a baby or show that they care for each other.

EXTRA INFO: Sex can be lots of different things. Sex or sexual intercourse is when the penis gets stiff, and they then put it into the vagina (or the female lets the male put their penis into the vagina). They also do other things like hug, kiss, and touch each other's bodies in a nice way. This is something that is just for adults.

What happens when you have sex?

Eventually your child will realize that adults don't just have sex to make babies. So, you can also start talking about how adults often kiss, hug, touch and engage in other sexual behaviors with one another to show caring for each other and to feel good.

There are lots of different ways to have sex. The main way that adults have sex to make a baby is when the penis goes into the vagina. They also do other things like hug, kiss, and touch each other's bodies in a nice way.

EXTRA INFO: Sex is something that most people do when they are grown up.

How do two females have sex?

You don't need to go into great detail here. Keep it simple!

There is more to sex than penises and vaginas. It is also about kissing, hugging, and touching each other's genitals. Gay (or lesbian) females can do all of this except for putting a penis in a vagina.

How do two males have sex?

You don't need to go into great detail here. Keep it simple!

There is more to sex than penises and vaginas. It is also about kissing, hugging, and touching each other's genitals. Gay males can do all of this except for putting a penis in a vagina.

Will I ever want to have sex?

One day you will, but not until puberty happens.

EXTRA INFO: During puberty, you will start to think about sex differently. This is because of your hormones.

Will I have sex one day?

Yes, you probably will have sex one day, but it won't be until you are an adult.

Why do people have sex?

Adults have sex for lots of different reasons. To make babies, to show their love for each other, and even for fun.

EXTRA INFO: Parents have sex and enjoy it. It is something that parents do.

Where do adults have sex?

Usually somewhere private, like in their bedroom.

EXTRA INFO: Sex is a private activity.

Do you have to lie down to have sex?

If you want to, you can. There are lots of different ways that adults can position their bodies to have sexual intercourse.

Do you have to be married to have sex?

The answer to this question depends on your personal beliefs.

Yes, in our family/church we believe that you need to be married to have sex.

OR

No, in our family we don't believe that you need to be married first. But we believe that you need to be an adult and in a loving and committed relationship first (or say what you believe in).

EXTRA INFO: But, physically, your grownup body is capable of having sex whether you are married or not.

Does it hurt to have sex?

Sometimes sex does hurt, but kids don't need to know about sexual pain yet.

No, sex doesn't hurt. Sex can feel really good.

What is an orgasm?

An orgasm is a really nice feeling that you can get during sex or when you touch your genitals in a nice way (masturbate).

What's an erection?

An erection is when the penis goes hard and erect.

EXTRA INFO: This happens when you have extra blood going into your penis.

EXTRA INFO: All males have erections, and they will start to have more of them as they get closer to puberty.

What does ejaculation mean?

Ejaculation is when semen, which contains sperm, comes out of the penis.

EXTRA INFO: The fluid comes out in little spurts, about a teaspoon in volume.

What is a virgin?

A virgin is someone who hasn't had sexual intercourse before.

How old do you have to be to have sex?

This answer depends on the law in the country and/or state that you live in. If you are unsure, just google 'legal age for sexual consent in (your state or country).'

The law says that you have to be (the legal age where you live). But in our family, we think that you shouldn't have sex until...' (you are married, in a loving and committed relationship, or whatever it is that you believe in).

What does sexy mean?

Sexy is a word that adults might use to describe someone that they think is attractive. It is a word that adults use.

You can add a value statement if you don't want your child to use this word, e.g. 'Sexy is not a word that we use in our family.'

What is oral sex?

Your child may hear other kids talking about oral sex and may be curious as to what it means. Remember to ask them why they are asking, just in case there is another reason for their question.

Oral sex is when people put their mouths on someone else's penis or vulva. This is something that is just for adults.

What is anal sex?

Your child may hear other kids talking about anal sex and may be curious as to what it means. Remember to ask them why they are asking, just in case there is another reason for their question.

Anal sex is when the penis goes into the anus (or bottom). This is something that is just for adults.

What is a condom?

A condom is something that people use when they don't want to have babies.

EXTRA INFO: It is like a long, skinny balloon, and it covers the penis.

Masturbation

You will need to talk with your child about what your family values and beliefs are on masturbation. Try to talk about this in a way that will not leave your child feeling shame and guilt. Kids just see it as a part of their body that feels good when you touch it. We now see it as a normal sexual behaviour that is not harmful. You can learn more about how to talk in this article - https://sexedrescue.com/child-masturbation/

Don't forget to remind your child that this is a private activity that should happen in a private place.

What is masturbation?

Masturbation is when you touch your penis or clitoris/vulva in a nice way and it feels good. People do it because it feels good.

EXTRA INFO: If a male is masturbating and their body has started to make sperm, they may ejaculate or come. This means that sticky white stuff called semen will come out of the end of their penis. There is usually a good feeling that goes with it called an orgasm.

Why do people masturbate?

Because it feels good.

EXTRA INFO: Usually because they have sexy feelings, i.e. tingly warm feelings in their body and genitals. Some people choose to masturbate when they have these feelings, but you don't have to.

EXTRA INFO: Some people masturbate a lot, and some just sometimes. Some don't masturbate at all.

How do you masturbate with a penis?

They may rub or pull on the penis. If their body has started to make sperm, they will usually ejaculate and reach orgasm.

How do you masturbate with a vulva?

They may touch or rub the vulva or clitoris. If they continue to rub and touch the clitoris and vulva, they might get a good feeling called an orgasm.

EXTRA INFO: An orgasm is a really nice warm tingly feeling around this area. It is a very strong feeling for a moment, and then it fades, leaving you with a warm, relaxed feeling.

Why does it feel nice when I touch my vulva/penis?

Sometimes it does feel nice when you touch yourself down there. That is just something that our bodies do and it means that your body is working properly.

EXTRA INFO: It feels nice because of your clitoris. The clitoris can feel nice when it is touched.

Love, attraction and gender identity

Regardless of your beliefs, children should be aware that sometimes we grow up and are attracted to the same sex and not the opposite sex. One in ten children grow up being attracted to the same sex, which means your child has a one in ten chance of being same-sex attracted.

All children need to know that sexual orientation is not a choice, all people deserve respect regardless of their sexual orientation, and who we are attracted to, whether it be females or males, is only a small part of who we are.

Try to discuss this topic with care and sensitivity, regardless of your beliefs. Sexual attraction is not a choice. If your child ends up being attracted to the same sex, how will they feel about it and will they feel safe talking to you about it?

If you explain this in a matter of fact way, your child won't find this confusing, especially if they are seeing same-sex couples within your community.

What does gay mean?

Gay can mean when a male loves a male or a female loves a female.

EXTRA INFO: Another word for it is homosexual.

Why are some people gay?

Being attracted to someone of the same sex is just something that happens. You can't stop it from happening. We don't really know why it happens.

Will I be gay?

You'll have to wait and see what happens as you get older. You will most probably be attracted to the opposite sex but you may be attracted to someone of the same sex or even both.

When will I know if I am gay?

Some kids know around puberty but for others, they may not know until they are in their late teens or are adults.

Who will I fall in love with?

You'll have to wait and see what happens as you get older. You will most probably be attracted to the opposite sex but you may be attracted to someone of the same sex or even both.

What does straight mean?

Straight means when males like females, and when females like males in a romantic way.

EXTRA INFO: Most people are straight, but some are gay. Who you are attracted to is only a small part of who you are.

What's a homosexual?

A homosexual is when a male likes other males, or a female likes other females, in a romantic way.

EXTRA INFO: Some of your friends in your class might be gay when they grow up. You could be, too. Who you are attracted to is only a small part of who you are, and you can't change it.

What's a heterosexual?

A heterosexual is when males like females and females like males in a romantic way.

What's a lesbian?

A lesbian is a female who likes other females in a romantic way.

EXTRA INFO: Some of your friends in your class might be lesbians when they grow up. You could be, too. Who you are attracted to is only a small part of who you are, and you can't change it.

What does trans or transgender mean?

Transgender is when your gender (boy or girl) doesn't match your sex (male or female). So, you might have a vulva but feel like a boy. Or you might have a penis and feel like a girl.

EXTRA INFO: Some people know this for sure from a very young age, and others don't find out for a while.

What does bisexual mean?

A bisexual is someone who likes both males and females in a romantic way.

EXTRA INFO: Some of your friends in your class might be bisexual when they grow up. You could be too. Who you are attracted to is only a small part of who you are and you can't change it.

What does asexual mean?

An asexual is someone who doesn't like males and females romantically.

EXTRA INFO: You and some of your friends in your class might be asexual when they grow up. You could be too. Who you are attracted to is only a small part of who you are and you can't change it.

What does Intersex mean?

You know when a baby is born and we call it a male or a female? Well, we make that decision because their genitals look male or female. Intersex is when we can't tell what the baby is by looking at its genitals.

EXTRA INFO: Intersex bodies are just a bit different to yours. They are still a kid just like you.

Bodies

> Learn more about teaching your child the names of their genitals in this article – https://sexedrescue.com/naming-private-parts/. You can find child-friendly diagrams to show your child here - https://sexedrescue.com/products/. And you can find books for talking to your child about their body here - https://sexedrescue.com/childrens-books-about-private-parts/.

Why does my penis go hard? (erection)

> You can let them know that erections have a sexual purpose when they are a bit older and curious about sexual intercourse. At the moment, though, it is just an amazing thing that their body can do.

That is what penises can do. It is called an erection.

EXTRA INFO: Why? It just shows that your penis is working properly.

Why is my friend's penis different?

Some penises are circumcised. This means that the skin on the end of their penis has been cut off. This means that the penis will look a little different at the end.

EXTRA INFO: Circumcision can happen for religious or cultural reasons, or because the foreskin can't stretch enough to be pushed back.

Why is my penis so small?

Penises come in all different sizes. Yours will grow bigger when you go through puberty. But for now, your penis is the right size for you.

What's an erection?

An erection is when your penis goes hard and erect.

EXTRA INFO: This happens when you have extra blood going into your penis.

EXTRA INFO: All males have erections and they will start to have more of them as they get closer to puberty.

Why are the testicles outside the body?

Sperm needs to be kept cooler than what your body temperature is. So, the sperm is stored outside of the body in the testicles, so that the sperm don't get too warm.

Do I have a uterus and eggs?

If your child asks why some people don't, just explain that most female bodies do, but that some female bodies don't. It is just something that happens when their body is being made inside their mommy's uterus.

Most females have a uterus and eggs, but some don't.

Do I have sperm?

Technically, not all males make sperm. They might have something wrong with the part of their body that makes sperm. Or they may be a transwoman (meaning they may still have male parts that make sperm).

No. Only grown up male bodies make sperm.

OR

No. Most males will make sperm when they are an adult, but some don't.

 You can access my FREE sex education course for parents at https://sexedrescue.com/ back-to-basics/

9 YEAR OLDS

Babies (and how they are made)

Some kids like to share this amazing information with their friends. So, it is a good idea to ask them not to. Try saying: 'Some parents like to talk to their own kids about where babies come from.'

Try to get into the habit of explaining what you think or believe when talking about love, sex and relationships. This is your opportunity to guide your child as they grow up, and to help them make healthy decisions around love, sex and relationships.

How are babies made?

A baby is made (or conceived) when sperm from the male joins with an egg/ovum from the female.

How does the sperm get to the egg?

If your child was made differently, you could explain the way that they were made. Refer to page 50 for an explanation.

The sperm leave the penis and go into the vagina. The sperm then find their way to the place where the egg is. The egg and the sperm then join together and grow into a baby.

EXTRA INFO: There are lots of different ways that the sperm and egg can get together. Sometimes they need help to get together.

How do the penis and vagina meet?

Kids sometimes get confused and think that the male removes their penis to do this.

The male and female have sex (sexual intercourse). They hold each other close, then the male's penis goes hard and is put into the vagina (or the female lets the male place their penis in the vagina). Sperm comes out of the penis into the vagina. The sperm then travels up inside the uterus, looking for an egg to fertilize (or turn into a baby). A baby may (or may not) happen.

Sex is something that is just for adults.

What other ways can a baby be made?

Refer to page 50 for explanations of the different ways babies can be made.

Sometimes the egg and sperm just can't get together. When this happens, the male and female need to see special doctors who collect their egg and sperm. The doctor will help the egg and sperm to join together and will then put it back inside the uterus, where it might grow into a baby.

How do two females make a baby?

A male will give one of the females some sperm, which will join with the egg and make a baby.

EXTRA INFO: The female might put the sperm into their vagina themself, or a special doctor might do this for them.

How do two males make a baby?

They will need to find a female who can grow a baby for them. They might use the egg from that person or another egg that someone has given them to use.

How is the egg made?

Females are born with their eggs already inside them.

EXTRA INFO: Eggs are found inside the ovaries.

How does the sperm find the egg?

The sperm are like tadpoles. They swim through the vagina and go up into the uterus, looking for an egg to fertilize.

How does the sperm fertilise the egg?

When the sperm find the egg, one of them will push and wiggle itself inside the egg.

EXTRA INFO: The egg closes up the hole, and then the egg and sperm become one cell – the beginning cell of a baby.

How is the egg made into a baby?

Once the sperm joins with the egg, it begins to divide into even more cells. This creates something called DNA, which is like a set of instructions on how the baby should grow.

How long does it take to make a baby?

The answer is based on how long it can take for the male to ejaculate with vaginal penetration.

Not very long. It can happen within a couple of minutes.

How long does it take for the sperm to find the egg?

Anywhere from half an hour to 5 days.

Do you have to have sex every time you want a baby?

You usually do, but there are also some other ways to make a baby.

EXTRA INFO: Sometimes you don't need to have sex to make a baby. Sometimes the people need help to get the egg and sperm together. This means that they need to get some special doctors to help the egg and sperm to join together to make a baby. This can happen for a lot of different medical reasons.

How many times do you need to have sex to make a baby?

You only need to have sex once to make a baby, but sometimes it takes more than one time to make a baby.

How old do you have to be to have a baby?

Males need to be making sperm before they can help to make a baby. So that could be anytime from the age of **13** or **14**.

Females need to be having their periods before they can become pregnant. So that could be anytime from the age of **10-11**.

You can also add a value statement about when you feel they should be having babies, e.g. 'In our family, we believe that you shouldn't have sex until...' (you are married, in a loving and committed relationship, are 16 or whatever it is that you believe in).

Can a male/man have a baby?

Technically, some men can have a baby, i.e. a transgender male may still have a uterus, which means they can become pregnant.

You need a uterus to grow a baby, so it is usually females (or women) that have babies.

EXTRA INFO: Sometimes a female doesn't feel like a girl on the inside. When they are grown up, they might dress and act like a man, even though they have a vagina. Or they might have a special operation that turns them into a male on the outside. If they leave the uterus (baby bag) in, it means that they could one day have a baby.

Sexual intercourse

Some kids like to share this amazing information with their friends. So, it is a good idea to ask them not to. Try saying: 'Some parents like to talk to their own kids about sexual intercourse.'

Your child will hear about sex at the playground, from their friends and through the media. This means that you have to be prepared for questions about sexual activities that are not age-appropriate, like bestiality (having sex with animals). Answering their questions will satisfy their curiosity and allow them to move on to something else, like, 'What's for dinner?' If you don't satisfy their curiosity, they may just go looking for an answer elsewhere, e.g. their friends or the internet.

If your child starts to ask questions about the different types of sexual behavior, it is usually a good idea to find out why they are asking the question. You could very casually say, 'Why are you asking that?' or, 'Where did you hear that word?'

When talking to kids about sex, you can add a value statement about the situations in which you believe sex should happen, e.g. 'In our family, we believe that you shouldn't have sex until...' (you are married, in a loving and committed relationship, are 16, or whatever it is that you believe in).

What is sex?

At first, kids are only curious about sex because they want to know how babies are made or they have heard whispers and giggles about this thing called sex. So, when we first start talking about sex (sexual intercourse), we can just talk about baby-making sex, i.e. sexual intercourse. Later on, we start adding in that there is a bit more to sex like hugging, kissing, etc. And that adults also have sex for other reasons as well. And we always remind kids that sex is something that adults do and that it is not for kids.

Sex is something that adults do when they want to make a baby or show that they care for each other.

EXTRA INFO: Sex can be lots of different things. Sex or sexual intercourse is when the penis gets stiff, and they then put it into the vagina (or the female lets the male put their penis into the vagina). They also do other things like hug, kiss, and touch each other's bodies in a nice way. This is something that is just for adults.

What happens when you have sex?

Eventually your child will realize that adults don't just have sex to make babies. So, you can also start talking about how adults often kiss, hug, touch and engage in other sexual behaviors with one another to show caring for each other and to feel good.

There are lots of different ways to have sex. The main way that adults have sex to make a baby is when the penis goes into the vagina. They also do other things like hug, kiss, and touch each other's bodies in a nice way.

EXTRA INFO: Sex is something that most people do when they are grown up.

How do two females have sex?

You don't need to go into great detail here. Keep it simple!

There is more to sex than penises and vaginas. It is also about kissing, hugging, and touching each other's genitals. Gay (or lesbian) females can do all of this except for putting a penis in a vagina.

How do two males have sex?

You don't need to go into great detail here. Keep it simple!

There is more to sex than penises and vaginas. It is also about kissing, hugging, and touching each other's genitals. Gay males can do all of this except for putting a penis in a vagina.

Will I ever want to have sex?

One day you will, but not until puberty happens.

EXTRA INFO: During puberty, you will start to think about sex differently. This is because of your hormones.

EXTRA INFO: You might find that you start thinking about someone in a new way. You may think about them a lot, have butterflies in your stomach when you meet and daydream about holding hands with them, hugging and kissing.

Will I have sex one day?

Yes, you probably will have sex one day, but it won't be until you are an adult.

Why do people have sex?

Adults have sex for lots of different reasons. To make babies, to show their love for each other, and even for fun.

EXTRA INFO: Parents have sex and enjoy it. It is something that parents do.

Where do adults have sex?

Usually somewhere private, like in their bedroom.

EXTRA INFO: Sex is a private activity.

Do you have to lie down to have sex?

If you want to, you can. There are lots of different ways that adults can position their bodies to have sexual intercourse.

Do you have to be married to have sex?

The answer to this question depends on your personal beliefs.

Yes, in our family/church, we believe that you need to be married to have sex.

OR

No, in our family we don't believe that you need to be married first. But we believe that you need to be an adult and in a loving and committed relationship first (or say what you believe in).

EXTRA INFO: But, physically, your grownup body is capable of having sex whether you are married or not.

Does it hurt to have sex?

Sometimes sex does hurt, but kids don't need to know about sexual pain yet.

No, sex doesn't hurt. Sex can feel really good.

EXTRA INFO: Your body is designed so that it doesn't usually hurt.

What is an orgasm?

An orgasm is a really nice feeling that you can get during sex or when you touch your genitals in a nice way (masturbate).

What's an erection?

An erection is when the penis goes hard and erect.

EXTRA INFO: This happens when you have extra blood going into your penis.

EXTRA INFO: All males have erections, and they will start to have more of them as they get closer to puberty.

What does ejaculation mean?

Ejaculation is when semen, which contains sperm, comes out of the penis.

EXTRA INFO: The fluid comes out in little spurts, about a teaspoon in volume.

What is a virgin?

A virgin is someone who hasn't had sexual intercourse before.

How old do you have to be to have sex?

This answer depends on the law in the country and/or state that you live in. If you are unsure, just google 'legal age for sexual consent in (your state or country).'

The law says that you have to be (the legal age where you live). But in our family, we think that you shouldn't have sex until...' (you are married, in a loving and committed relationship, or whatever it is that you believe in).

Other sexual activities

This section provides age-appropriate explanations about topics that are NOT age-appropriate, i.e. it isn't really stuff that kids need to know (just yet).

So, why is it in here? Because kids hear about this sort of sex stuff at a very young age! And this is the sort of stuff that kids of this age are starting to talk about.

We need to help our kids to process and make sense of this sex stuff. If we can answer their questions and satisfy their curiosity, they are more likely to move onto the next great mystery in their life, like why is there no bread in the fridge!

The main thing is to emphasise that this is for adults (not for kids) and that this stuff isn't everyday sex stuff. You see a lot of this stuff in porn, but porn is made-up sex and not necessarily what happens in most bedrooms.

And don't forget to check why they are asking!

What is oral sex?

Your child may hear other kids talking about oral sex and may be curious as to what it means. Remember to ask them why they are asking, just in case there is another reason for their question.

Oral sex is when people put their mouths on someone else's penis or vulva. This is something that is just for adults.

What is anal sex?

Your child may hear other kids talking about anal sex and may be curious as to what it means. Remember to ask them why they are asking, just in case there is another reason for their question.

Anal sex is when the penis goes into the anus (or bottom). This is something that is just for adults.

What's a fetish?

A fetish is when a person needs something, like a shoe, a car or another object, to feel sexy.

EXTRA INFO: There are lots of different fetishes, and it depends on the person as to what they like.

Why do people like to watch each other have sex? (voyeurism)

Some people like to watch other people have sex. The people having sex will know that they are being watched.

A peeping tom is when some people, usually males, like to peep on females when they are naked or having sex. They usually don't know that someone is watching them unless they catch them peeping.

EXTRA INFO: This is a crime and not the sort of thing that kids should be doing.

Prostitution (Paid sex)

What is a prostitute?

A prostitute is someone who gets paid to have sex with other people.

EXTRA INFO: They are also called a sex worker or a prostitute. There are also some other names that people use for them.

EXTRA INFO: A person will pay the prostitute to have sexual intercourse or to do other sex things with them.

EXTRA INFO: Prostitutes are both males and females, and they may have sex with the opposite sex and/or the same sex.

Why do people pay for sex?

I don't really know. They may pay for sex because they don't have a sexual partner of their own or their partner may not be able to have sex. People pay for sex for their own reasons.

Why do people do that for a job?

> The reasons you give your child will be heavily influenced by your own personal beliefs but try to keep an open mind and to not judge.

People do this work because it is a job, i.e. they do it for the money. They usually don't know the person who is paying them for sex.

EXTRA INFO: They might enjoy this type of work or helping people, or they may think that it is the best way that they can earn money. Some do it because they are addicted to drugs and they can earn enough money to pay for their drugs. Or because they have no other way to earn money.

Bestiality (Sex with animals)

Do people have sex with animals?

> Pornography has changed and animal porn is now very easy to find. So, you need to be prepared to be asked about it, just in case your child finds it or hears their peers talking about it.

Yes, some people do have sex with animals.

EXTRA INFO: It is wrong to have sex with animals.

EXTRA INFO: Bestiality is a crime and there are laws against having sex with animals. This is not something for kids to do.

EXTRA INFO: If you find this sort of stuff online, you need to come and tell me. You won't get into trouble.

Why do people do it?

They might do it just for fun or to try something different. I don't really know why they do it but they shouldn't have sex with animals.

EXTRA INFO: You often see bestiality in porn. Porn sex isn't real, everyday sex. This is not something for kids to do.

EXTRA INFO: If you find this sort of stuff online, you need to come and tell me. You won't get into trouble.

How do people do it?

The female might let the animal put its penis in their vagina or to lick their vulva. The male might put their penis in the animal's anus or vagina or let it lick their penis.

Group sex (Sex with more than one person)

What is group sex?

Group sex is when three or more people might decide to have sex together.

Why do people do it?

They might do it just for fun or to try something different. I don't really know why they do it.

EXTRA INFO: You often see this stuff in porn. Porn sex isn't real, everyday sex.

EXTRA INFO: If you find this sort of stuff online, you need to come and tell me. You won't get into trouble.

Sexual aids

What is a sex toy?

They aren't real toys like what you play with. They are just things that grownups can buy that they might use when they are having sex.

EXTRA INFO: Some sex toys are like a toy plastic penis or vagina. Some vibrate. There are lots of different things that people can buy if they want to.

Why do people use them? (sex toys)

People use them to masturbate by themselves or with their partner.

They use them for lots of different reasons. They might think that it makes sex more interesting or fun.

EXTRA INFO: Not all people use sex toys. It is a decision that people make on their own or with their partner.

EXTRA INFO: This is a grown-up thing and not for kids.

Why do people like to dress up during sex? (role-play/ lingerie)

Some grownups like to play games during sex. They might dress up or use special gear.

EXTRA INFO: If you find this sort of stuff online, you need to come and tell me. You won't get into trouble.

Bondage & Discipline (B&D)

What is B&D?

That's a type of sex that some adults do. One person will be really bossy and the other person will do what they tell them to do.

Why do people like to do it?

I don't know. It is just something that some people like to do.

EXTRA INFO: It isn't the sort of sex that people do every day, though.

EXTRA INFO: If you find this sort of stuff online, you need to come and tell me. You won't get into trouble.

Sadomasochism (S&M)

What is S&M?

S&M is a game where one person wants to be hurt a little during sex. They decide how they want to be hurt, how much and their partner hurts them a little.

EXTRA INFO: Even though they're called a game, this is a grown-up thing and not for kids.

EXTRA INFO: If you find this sort of stuff online, you need to come and tell me. You won't get into trouble.

Why do people like to hurt each other during sex?

To a child, listening to sex can sound like someone is being hurt. So, check first to see what they are referring to? Are they referring to everyday sex or the sort of rough sex that can happen in movies and on the internet?

I don't know. It is just something that some people like to do.

Pole dancing

What's pole dancing?

That's a special sort of dancing that some people do.

EXTRA INFO: It is dancing that is just for grownups and not for kids.

Why do they dance like that?

It is special sexy dancing and some people like to watch it happen. Some people do it for a job but some do it for fun or to keep fit.

EXTRA INFO: Some grownups think that pole dancing isn't a very nice thing to do. So, you might hear them, or other kids, laughing and joking about it.

Stripping

What's stripping?

It is when people take their clothes off while they dance to music.

Why do people do it?

It can be a job for some people as they get paid to do it.

Masturbation

You will need to talk with your child about what your family values and beliefs are on masturbation. Try to talk about this in a way that will not leave your child feeling shame and guilt. Kids just see it as a part of their body that feels good when you touch it. We now see it as a normal sexual behaviour that is not harmful. You can learn more about how to talk in this article - https://sexedrescue.com/child-masturbation/

What is masturbation?

Masturbation is when you touch your penis or clitoris/vulva in a nice way and it feels good. People do it because it can feel nice.

EXTRA INFO: If a male is masturbating and their body has started to make sperm, they may ejaculate or come. This means that sticky white stuff called semen will come out of the end of their penis. There is usually a good feeling that goes with it called an orgasm.

Why do people masturbate?

Because it can feel nice and they like how it makes them feel.

EXTRA INFO: Usually because they have sexy feelings, i.e. tingly warm feelings in their body and genitals. Some people choose to masturbate when they have these feelings.

EXTRA INFO: Some people masturbate a lot, and some just sometimes. Some don't masturbate at all.

How do you masturbate with a penis?

They may rub or pull on the penis. If their body has started to make sperm, they will usually ejaculate and reach orgasm.

How do masturbate with a vulva?

They may touch or rub the vulva or clitoris. If they continue to rub and touch the clitoris and vulva, they might get a good feeling called an orgasm.

What is an orgasm?

An orgasm is a really nice feeling that you can get during sex or when you touch your genitals in a nice way (masturbate).

An orgasm is a really nice warm, tingly feeling around this area. It is a very strong feeling for a moment, and then it fades, leaving you with a warm, relaxed feeling.

Love, attraction and gender identity

You will find age-appropriate questions and answers about love and attraction and gender identity on page 108.

Penises, erections and wet dreams

You can find child-friendly diagrams to show your child here - https://sexedrescue. com/products/. And you can find books for talking to your child about their body here - https://sexedrescue.com/childrens-books-about-private-parts/.

What's an erection?

An erection is when the penis goes hard and erect.

EXTRA INFO: This happens when there is extra blood going into the penis.

EXTRA INFO: All males have erections and they will start to have more of them as they get closer to puberty.

What does ejaculation mean?

Ejaculation is when semen and sperm come out of the penis.

EXTRA INFO: The fluid comes out in little spurts, about a teaspoon in volume.

What's the difference between sperm and semen?

Sperm is made by your testicles during puberty and is needed to make a baby. Semen is the whitish fluid that carries the sperm.

Why is my friend's penis different?

Some penises are circumcised. This means that the skin on the end of their penis has been cut off. This means that the penis will look a little different at the end.

EXTRA INFO: Circumcision can happen for religious or cultural reasons, or because the foreskin can't stretch enough to be pushed back.

Why is my penis so small?

Penises come in all different sizes. Yours will grow bigger when you go through puberty. But for now, your penis is the right size for you.

Do I have sperm?

Technically, not all males make sperm. They might have something wrong with the part of their body that makes sperm.

No. Only grown up male bodies make sperm.

OR

No. Most males will make sperm when they are an adult, but some don't.

Why are the testicles outside the body?

Sperm need to be kept cooler than what your body temperature is. The sperm is stored outside of the body in the testicles so that the sperm don't get too warm.

You can access my FREE sex education course for parents at https://sexedrescue.com/back-to-basics/

10 YEAR OLDS

Babies (and how they are made)

Try to get into the habit of explaining what you think or believe when talking about love, sex and relationships. This is your opportunity to guide your child as they grow up, and to help them make healthy decisions around love, sex and relationships.

How are babies made?

A baby is made (or conceived) when sperm from the male joins with an egg/ovum from the female.

How does the sperm get to the egg?

The sperm leave the penis and go into the vagina. The sperm then find their way to the place where the egg is. The egg and the sperm then join together and grow into a baby.

EXTRA INFO: There are lots of different ways that the sperm and egg can get together. Sometimes they need help to get together.

How do the penis and vagina meet?

Kids sometimes get confused and think that the male removes their penis to do this.

The male and female have sex (sexual intercourse). They hold each other close, then the male's penis goes hard and is put into the vagina (or the female lets the male place their penis in the vagina). Sperm

134

comes out of the penis into the vagina. The sperm then travels up inside the uterus, looking for an egg to fertilize (or turn into a baby). A baby may (or may not) happen.

Sex is something that is just for adults.

What other ways can a baby be made?

Sometimes the egg and sperm just can't get together. When this happens, the male and female need to see special doctors who collect their egg and sperm. The doctor will help the egg and sperm to join together, and they will then put it back inside the uterus, where it might grow into a baby.

How do two females make a baby?

A male will give one of the females some sperm, which will join with the egg and make a baby.

EXTRA INFO: The female might put the sperm into their vagina themself, or a special doctor might do this for them.

How do two males make a baby?

They will need to find a female who can grow a baby for them. They might use the egg from that person or another egg that someone has given them to use.

How is the egg made?

Females are born with their eggs already inside them.

EXTRA INFO: Eggs are found inside the ovaries.

How does the sperm find the egg?

The sperm are like tadpoles. They swim through the vagina and go up into the uterus, looking for an egg to fertilize.

How does the sperm fertilize the egg?

When the sperm find the egg, one of them will push and wiggle itself inside the egg.

EXTRA INFO: The egg closes up the hole, and then the egg and sperm become one cell – the beginning cell of a baby.

How is the egg made into a baby?

Once the sperm joins with the egg, it begins to divide into even more cells. This creates something called DNA, which is like a set of instructions on how the baby should grow.

How long does it take to make a baby?

This answer is based on how long it can take for the male to ejaculate with vaginal penetration.

Not very long. It can happen within a couple of minutes.

How long does it take for the sperm to find the egg?

Anywhere from half an hour to 5 days.

Do you have to have sex every time you want a baby?

You usually do, but there are also some other ways to make a baby.

EXTRA INFO: Sometimes you don't need to have sex to make a baby. Sometimes the people need help to get the egg and sperm together. This means that they need to get some special doctors to help the egg and sperm to join together to make a baby. This can happen for a lot of different medical reasons.

How many times do you need to have sex to make a baby?

You only need to have sex once to make a baby, but sometimes it takes more than one time to make a baby.

How old do you have to be to have a baby?

Males need to be making sperm before they can help to make a baby. So that could be anytime from the age of **13** or **14**.

Females need to be having their periods before they can become pregnant. So that could be anytime from the age of **10-11**.

You can also add a value statement about when you feel they should be having babies, e.g. 'In our family, we believe that you shouldn't have sex until...' (you are married, in a loving and committed relationship, are 16 or whatever it is that you believe in).

Sexual intercourse

Some kids like to share this amazing information with their friends. So, it is a good idea to ask them not to. Try saying: 'Some parents like to talk to their own kids about sexual intercourse.'

Your child will hear about sex at the playground, from their friends and through the media. This means that you have to be prepared for questions about sexual activities that are not age-appropriate, like bestiality (having sex with animals). Answering their questions will satisfy their curiosity and allow them to move on to something else, like, 'What's for dinner?' If you don't satisfy their curiosity, they may just go looking for an answer elsewhere, e.g. their friends or the internet.

If your child starts to ask questions about the different types of sexual behavior, it is usually a good idea to find out why they are asking the question. You could very casually say, 'Why are you asking that?' or, 'Where did you hear that word?'

You can add a value statement about the situations in which you believe sex should happen, e.g. 'In our family, we believe that you shouldn't have sex until...' (you are married, in a loving and committed relationship, are 16, or whatever it is that you believe in).

What is sex?

At first, kids are only curious about sex because they want to know how babies are made or they have heard whispers and giggles about this thing called sex. So, when we first start talking about sex (sexual intercourse), we can just talk about baby-making sex, i.e. sexual intercourse. Later on, we start adding in that there is a bit more to sex like hugging, kissing, etc. And that adults also have sex for other reasons as well. And we always remind kids that sex is something that adults do and that it is not for kids.

Sex or sexual intercourse is something that adults do when they want to make a baby or show that they care for each other.

They usually find somewhere private, like their bedroom, and will take their clothes off. They will hug and kiss and touch each other's bodies all over. The penis will go stiff and they will push it inside the vagina (or the female will let the male push their penis into the vagina). They will then move together until the male ejaculates.

EXTRA INFO: Adults can choose whether they want to have a baby or not.

What happens when you have sex?

Eventually your child will realize that adults don't just have sex to make babies. So, you can also start talking about how adults often kiss, hug, touch and engage in other sexual behaviors with one another to show caring for each other and to feel good.

There are lots of different ways to have sex. The main way that adults have sex to make a baby is when the penis goes vagina. They also do other things like hug, kiss, and touch each other's bodies in a nice way.

EXTRA INFO: Sex is something that most people do when they are grown up.

How do two females have sex?

You don't need to go into great detail here. Keep it simple!

There is more to sex than penises and vaginas. It is also about kissing, hugging, and touching each other's genitals. Gay (or lesbian) females can do all of this except for putting a penis in a vagina.

How do two males have sex?

You don't need to go into great detail here. Keep it simple!

There is more to sex than penises and vaginas. It is also about kissing, hugging, and touching each other's genitals. Gay males can do all of this except for putting a penis in a vagina.

Will I ever want to have sex?

One day you will, but not until puberty happens.

EXTRA INFO: During puberty, you will start to think about sex differently. This is because of your hormones.

EXTRA INFO: You might find that you start thinking about someone in a new way. You may think about them a lot, have butterflies in your stomach when you meet and daydream about holding hands with them, hugging and kissing.

Will I have sex one day?

Yes, you probably will have sex one day, but it won't be until you are an adult.

When will I want to have sex?

Kids sometimes struggle to understand why they might ever want to have sex one day. One way to explain this is to talk about our 'sex switch.' That switch doesn't get turned on until puberty. Once the switch is turned on, it slowly starts to rewire your brain so that you see sex as something that you want to do instead of something that is weird or gross.

You won't be interested in having sex until puberty happens. Once your body starts making hormones, you will start to think about sex and about people in a different way.

EXTRA INFO: Most people don't just have sex with a complete stranger. They usually start off by getting to know another person first, then become friends. The couple will usually hold hands, hug, cuddle and kiss before they get to the sex part.

Why do people have sex?

Adults have sex for lots of different reasons. To make babies, to show their love for each other, and even for fun.

EXTRA INFO: Parents have sex and enjoy it. It is something that parents do.

EXTRA INFO: A lot of things usually happen before a relationship becomes sexual. The two people usually start off being friends first and will hold hands, hug, cuddle and kiss before they get to the sex part.

Where do adults have sex?

Usually somewhere private, like in their bedroom.

EXTRA INFO: Sex is a private activity.

Do you have to lie down to have sex?

If you want to, you can. There are lots of different ways that adults can position their bodies to have sexual intercourse.

Do you have to be married to have sex?

The answer to this question depends on your personal beliefs.

Yes, in our family/church, we believe that you need to be married to have sex.

OR

No, in our family, we don't believe that you need to be married first. But we believe that you need to be an adult and in a loving and committed relationship first (or say what you believe in).

EXTRA INFO: But, physically, your grownup body is capable of having sex whether you are married or not.

Does it hurt to have sex?

Sometimes sex does hurt, but kids don't need to know about sexual pain yet.

No, sex doesn't hurt. Sex can feel really good.

EXTRA INFO: Your body is designed so that it doesn't usually hurt.

What is an orgasm?

An orgasm is a really nice feeling that you can get during sex or when you touch your genitals in a nice way (masturbate).

EXTRA INFO: Males usually ejaculate when they reach orgasm or climax.

What's an erection?

An erection is when the penis goes hard and erect.

EXTRA INFO: This happens because there is extra blood going into the penis.

EXTRA INFO: All males have erections, and they will start to have more of them as they get closer to puberty.

What does ejaculation mean?

Ejaculation is when semen, which contains sperm, comes out of the penis.

EXTRA INFO: The fluid comes out in little spurts, about a teaspoon in volume.

What is a virgin?

A virgin is someone who hasn't had sexual intercourse before.

How old do you have to be to have sex?

This answer depends on the law in the country and/or state that you live in. If you are unsure, just google 'legal age for sexual consent in (your state or country).'

The law says that you have to be (the legal age where you live). But in our family, we think that you shouldn't have sex until...' (you are married, in a loving and committed relationship, or whatever it is that you believe in).

Other sexual activities

Thanks to the oversexualised world we live in (and the porn that kids are exposed to), kids are hearing not just about baby-making-sex, but about all the other types of sex that can happen. Things like anal and oral sex, sexual fetishes, prostitution, bestiality, group sex, sex toys, B&D, S&M, pole dancing, stripping and more. So, you can find age-appropriate answers for questions about these things on page 122.

Masturbation

You will need to talk with your child about what your family values and beliefs are on masturbation. Try to talk about this in a way that will not leave your child feeling shame and guilt. Kids just see it as a part of their body that feels good when you touch it. We now see it as a normal sexual behaviour that is not harmful. You can learn more about how to talk in this article - https://sexedrescue.com/child-masturbation/

What is masturbation?

Masturbation is when you touch your penis or clitoris/vulva in a nice way and it feels good. People do it because it feels good.

EXTRA INFO: If a male is masturbating and their body has started to make sperm, they may ejaculate or come. This means that sticky white stuff called semen will come out of the end of their penis. There is usually a good feeling that goes with it called an orgasm.

Why do people masturbate?

Because it feels good.

EXTRA INFO: Usually because they have sexy feelings, i.e. tingly warm feelings in their body and genitals. Some people choose to masturbate when they have these feelings.

EXTRA INFO: Some people masturbate a lot, and some just sometimes. Some don't masturbate at all.

How do you masturbate with a penis?

They may rub or pull on the penis. If their body has started to make sperm, they will usually ejaculate and reach orgasm.

How do masturbate with a vulva?

They may touch or rub the vulva or clitoris. If they continue to rub and touch the clitoris and vulva, they might get a good feeling called an orgasm.

What is an orgasm?

An orgasm is a really nice feeling that you can get during sex or when you touch your genitals in a nice way (masturbate).

An orgasm is a really nice warm, tingly feeling around this area. It is a very strong feeling for a moment, and then it fades, leaving you with a warm, relaxed feeling.

Love, attraction and gender identity

You will find age-appropriate questions and answers about love and attraction and gender identity on page 108.

Contraception

Kids can understand that there are ways to stop a pregnancy from happening or continuing. They don't need to know about the details at this age as it really isn't relevant until they start thinking about sex as something that they might want to do.

What is contraception?

Contraception is something that you can do to prevent pregnancy.

EXTRA INFO: It is usually something that females use.

EXTRA INFO: Contraception can be many different things. It could be a tablet that is taken each day, or an injection every few months, an implant that goes into the arm, something that is inside the vagina or uterus or an operation.

If your religion doesn't believe in contraception, you will need to talk about natural methods instead. You could try saying: 'Our faith doesn't believe in contraception. So, to try to prevent pregnancy, we have sex when we are less likely to fall pregnant.'

Can males use contraception?

Yes, they can. They can use something that will stop a female from becoming pregnant.

EXTRA INFO: Males can wear a condom to stop their sperm from going into the vagina. (A condom is like a special balloon that fits over the penis.)

EXTRA INFO: By the time you are an adult, there may even be an injection or a tablet that men can take. Some men can have a special operation that will stop their sperm from coming out (vasectomy).

What is a condom?

A condom is something that people use when they don't want to have babies.

EXTRA INFO: It is like a long, skinny balloon, and it covers the penis.

What is a vasectomy?

A special operation for males where the tube that carries the sperm from the testicles is cut and tied up so that no sperm can come out. Semen will still come out but there will be no sperm in it.

EXTRA INFO: The male will still make sperm but they will just get absorbed into their body, instead of coming out of the penis.

What is a tubal ligation?

A special operation for females where the tube that carries the egg is cut and tied so that the egg can't come out.

EXTRA INFO: The female will still release an egg each month but it will just get absorbed into their body.

What is an abortion?

An abortion (or termination) is when a person is pregnant and they can choose to have the pregnancy stopped.

EXTRA INFO: They might do this because there is something wrong with them or the baby or because they don't want to have a baby.

EXTRA INFO: They might have a special operation or take medicine that will make the pregnancy terminate (or finish).

If you are against terminating a pregnancy, you need to tell your child and explain why, e.g. 'I don't believe that people should have abortions because...'

Sexually Transmitted Infections (or STIs)

Kids will hear about STIs (sexually transmitted infections) and possibly even see the posters promoting screenings when using public bathrooms. They don't need to know all the details yet, as it isn't relevant. But it is important that they know that infections can be spread through sexual activity.

What is an STI?

If someone has germs or viruses in their vagina, penis or blood, they can pass the germs on to the person that they are having sex with. This means that the person that they are having sex with can get sick, too.

EXTRA INFO: Some STIs can last a lifetime. Most STIs are treatable, but some aren't.

EXTRA INFO: There are many different kinds of STIs. Some of them include genital warts, herpes, gonorrhoea, chlamydia, syphilis, HIV, hepatitis A, B and C, and pubic lice.

What is safe sex?

Safe sex means ways of having sex without getting any infections or becoming pregnant.

EXTRA INFO: It can mean a way to have sex where you don't get semen or vaginal fluid onto the other person's body.

EXTRA INFO: Condoms are one way of having safe sex.

Penises, erections and wet dreams

Learn more about teaching your child the names of their genitals in this article – https://sexedrescue.com/naming-private-parts/. You can also find child-friendly diagrams to use with your child here - https://sexedrescue.com/products/.

Why is my friend's penis different?

Some penises are circumcised. This means that the skin on the end of their penis has been cut off. This means that the penis will look a little different at the end.

EXTRA INFO: Circumcision can happen for religious or cultural reasons, or because the foreskin can't stretch enough to be pushed back.

Why is my penis so small?

Penises come in all different sizes. Yours will grow bigger when you go through puberty. But for now, your penis is the right size for you.

What's an erection?

An erection is when your penis goes hard and erect.

EXTRA INFO: This happens when you have extra blood going into your penis.

EXTRA INFO: All males have erections and they will start to have more of them as they get closer to puberty.

What is sperm?

Sperm is the male reproductive cell and is needed to make a baby.

What is semen?

Semen is the liquid that carries the sperm.

EXTRA INFO: Semen is sticky, cloudy (not clear) and whitish in colour.

EXTRA INFO: Its job is to keep the sperm healthy.

Do I have sperm?

Most males will one day make sperm when they go through puberty, usually when they are between **12-14** years old.

When will I start to make sperm?

Males usually start to make sperm when they are **13** and a half. Some will make it sooner and some will make it later.

What's a 'wet dream'?

A wet dream is when you ejaculate semen and sperm during your sleep. You might wake up when it happens, or you may just find a wet patch on your pants or sheets the next morning.

EXTRA INFO: Wet dreams only happen once your body starts to make semen and sperm.

EXTRA INFO: This is a normal thing to happen to males. Some males have many; some males, not as many; and some males never have a wet dream.

Can females have wet dreams?

Yes, they can have wet dreams too.

Puberty

Don't forget to remind your child that we all start puberty at different times. And that our bodies will all change differently. Breasts, penises and our bodies come in all different shapes and sizes. Reassure them that they are normal.

What is puberty?

Puberty is when your body changes from being a child to an adult body.

Why does puberty happen?

To get your body ready so that you can have a baby when you are all grown up.

What makes puberty happen?

Your body makes special chemicals called hormones. They make your body begin to change.

When will puberty happen?

Everybody is different. For most people it can be from as young as **8** or as late as **16.**

EXTRA INFO: Your body will start to change when it is the right size and shape for you.

EXTRA INFO: Females go through puberty first. Males usually start 2 years later.

How do I know when puberty is going to happen?

You won't really know until you start to see some changes in your own body. Everyone starts puberty at a different time. Some of your friends will start earlier, later or at the same time as you.

What changes happen to female bodies?

- breasts begin to grow and develop
- hips become wider
- thighs and bottoms become more rounded
- armpit and pubic hair begin to grow
- body odour becomes stronger
- uterus, vagina and ovaries grow and begin to release eggs
- menstruation (periods) starts

What changes happen to male bodies?

- body shape becomes taller, heavier and more muscular, shoulders and chest broaden
- their voice begins to deepen
- armpit and pubic hair begin to grow
- body odour becomes stronger
- erections start happening more frequently (sometimes when you least expect them) and wet dreams occur more frequently
- penis, testicles and scrotum start to grow larger

Why do I get white stuff on my underpants?

That is something that happens to your body as you start puberty. We call it vaginal discharge and it is the vagina's way of cleaning itself.

What's a period?

A period is a small amount of blood that comes out of a vagina every month.

EXTRA INFO: Each month, the body prepares itself in case a baby is made. The uterus makes a special lining which is ready for the fertilised egg to land on, which is where it will then grow into a baby. If a baby doesn't happen, the lining is no longer needed. The lining then comes out through the vagina as menstrual blood or a period. Your body will do this each month.

EXTRA INFO: This cycle will keep on happening until your hormones tell it to stop.

Why do people have periods?

It is a part of the what the body does, to get ready for falling pregnant. Each month the uterus makes a special lining of blood to grow a baby onto. When a baby isn't made, the special lining isn't needed, so it comes out of the vagina as blood.

When will I get my period?

Some people can be as young as **8** or as old as **16** before they start their period.

 You can access my FREE sex education course for parents at https://sexedrescue.com/back-to-basics/

11 YEAR OLDS

Babies (and how they are made)

How are babies made?

A baby is made (or conceived) when sperm from the male joins with an egg/ovum from the female.

How does the sperm get to the egg?

The sperm leave the penis and go into the vagina. The sperm then find their way to the place where the egg is. The egg and the sperm then join together and grow into a baby.

EXTRA INFO: There are lots of different ways that the sperm and egg can get together. Sometimes they need help to get together.

How do the penis and vagina meet?

Kids sometimes get confused and think that the male removes their penis to do this.

The male and female have sex (sexual intercourse). They hold each other close, the male's penis goes hard, and is put into the vagina (or the female lets the male place their penis in the vagina). Sperm comes

153

out of the penis into the vagina. The sperm then travels up inside the uterus, looking for an egg to fertilize (or turn into a baby). A baby may (or may not) happen.

Sex is something that is just for adults.

What other ways can a baby be made?

Sometimes the egg and sperm just can't get together. When this happens, the male and female need to see special doctors who collect their egg and sperm. The doctor will help the egg and sperm to join together, and they will then put it back inside the uterus, where it might grow into a baby.

How do two females make a baby?

A male will give one of the females some sperm, which will join with the egg and make a baby.

EXTRA INFO: The female might put the sperm into their vagina themself, or a special doctor might do this for them.

How do two males make a baby?

They will need to find a female who can grow a baby for them. They might use the egg from that person or another egg that someone has given them to use.

How is the egg made?

Females are born with their eggs already inside them.

EXTRA INFO: Eggs are found inside the ovaries.

How does the sperm find the egg?

The sperm are like tadpoles. They swim through the vagina and go up into the uterus, looking for an egg to fertilize.

How does the sperm fertilize the egg?

When the sperm find the egg, one of them will push and wiggle itself inside the egg.

EXTRA INFO: The egg closes up the hole, and then the egg and sperm become one cell – the beginning cell of a baby.

How is the egg made into a baby?

Once the sperm joins with the egg, it begins to divide into even more cells. This creates something called DNA, which is like a set of instructions on how the baby should grow.

How long does it take to make a baby?

This answer is based on how long it can take for the male to ejaculate with vaginal penetration.

Not very long. It can happen within a couple of minutes.

How long does it take for the sperm to find the egg?

Anywhere from half an hour to 5 days.

Do you have to have sex every time you want a baby?

You usually do, but there are also some other ways to make a baby.

EXTRA INFO: Sometimes you don't need to have sex to make a baby. Sometimes the people need help to get the egg and sperm together. This means that they need to get some special doctors to help the egg and sperm to join together to make a baby. This can happen for a lot of different medical reasons.

How many times do you need to have sex to make a baby?

You only need to have sex once to make a baby, but sometimes it takes more than one time to make a baby.

How old do you have to be to have a baby?

Males need to be making sperm before they can help to make a baby. So that could be anytime from the age of **13** or **14**.

Females need to be having their periods before they can become pregnant. So that could be anytime from the age of **10-11**.

You can also add a value statement about when you feel they should be having babies, e.g. 'In our family, we believe that you shouldn't have sex until...' (you are married, in a loving and committed relationship, are 16 or whatever it is that you believe in).

Sexual intercourse

Your child will have already heard about sex at the playground, from their friends and through the media. This means that you have to be prepared for questions about sexual activities that are not age-appropriate, like bestiality (having sex with animals). Answering their questions will satisfy their curiosity and allow them to move on to something else, like, 'What's for dinner?' If you don't satisfy their curiosity, they may just go looking for an answer elsewhere, e.g. their friends or the internet.

If your child starts to ask questions about the different types of sexual behavior, it is usually a good idea to find out why they are asking the question. You could very casually say, 'Why are you asking that?' or, 'Where did you hear that word?'

When talking to kids about sex, you can add a value statement about the situations in which you believe sex should happen, e.g. 'In our family, we believe that you shouldn't have sex until...' (you are married, in a loving and committed relationship, are 16, or whatever it is that you believe in).

What is sex?

At first, kids are only curious about sex because they want to know how babies are made or they have heard whispers and giggles about this thing called sex. So, when we first start talking about sex (sexual intercourse), we can just talk about baby-making sex, i.e. sexual intercourse. Later on, we start adding in that there is a bit more to sex like hugging, kissing, etc. And that adults also have sex for other reasons as well. And we always remind kids that sex is something that adults do and that it is not for kids.

Sex or sexual intercourse is something that adults do when they want to make a baby or show that they care for each other.

They usually find somewhere private, like their bedroom, and will take their clothes off. They will hug and kiss and touch each other's bodies all over. The penis will go stiff and they will push it inside the vagina (or the female will let the male push their penis into the vagina). They will then move together until the male ejaculates.

EXTRA INFO: Adults can choose whether they want to have a baby or not.

What happens when you have sex?

Eventually your child will realize that adults don't just have sex to make babies. So, you can also start talking about how adults often kiss, hug, touch and engage in other sexual behaviors with one another to show caring for each other and to feel good.

There are lots of different ways to have sex. The main way that adults have sex to make a baby is when the penis goes vagina. They also do other things like hug, kiss, and touch each other's bodies in a nice way.

EXTRA INFO: Sex is something that most people do when they are grown up.

How do two females have sex?

> You don't need to go into great detail here. Keep it simple!

There is more to sex than penises and vaginas. It is also about kissing, hugging, and touching each other's genitals. Gay (or lesbian) females can do all of this except for putting a penis in a vagina.

How do two males have sex?

> You don't need to go into great detail here. Keep it simple!

There is more to sex than penises and vaginas. It is also about kissing, hugging, and touching each other's genitals. Gay males can do all of this except for putting a penis in a vagina.

Will I ever want to have sex?

One day you will, but not until puberty happens.

EXTRA INFO: During puberty, you will start to think about sex differently. This is because of your hormones.

Will I have sex one day?

Yes, you probably will have sex one day, but it won't be until you are an adult.

When will I want to have sex?

> Kids sometimes struggle to understand why they might ever want to have sex one day. One way to explain this is to talk about our 'sex switch.' That switch doesn't get turned on until puberty. Once the switch is turned on, it slowly starts to

rewire your brain so that you see sex as something that you want to do instead of something that is weird or gross.

You won't be interested in having sex until puberty happens. Once your body starts making hormones, you will start to think about sex and about people in a different way.

EXTRA INFO: Most people don't just have sex with a complete stranger. They usually start off by getting to know another person first, then become friends. The couple will usually hold hands, hug, cuddle and kiss before they get to the sex part.

Why do people have sex?

Adults have sex for lots of different reasons. To make babies, to show their love for each other, and even for fun.

EXTRA INFO: Parents have sex and enjoy it. It is something that parents do.

EXTRA INFO: A lot of things usually happen before a relationship becomes sexual. The two people usually start off being friends first and will hold hands, hug, cuddle and kiss before they get to the sex part.

Where do adults have sex?

Usually somewhere private, like in their bedroom.

EXTRA INFO: Sex is a private activity.

Do you have to lie down to have sex?

If you want to, you can. There are lots of different ways that adults can position their bodies to have sexual intercourse.

Do you have to be married to have sex?

The answer to this question depends on your personal beliefs.

Yes, in our family/church we believe that you need to be married to have sex.

OR

No, in our family we don't believe that you need to be married first. But we believe that you need to be an adult and in a loving and committed relationship first (or say what you believe in).

EXTRA INFO: But, physically, your grownup body is capable of having sex whether you are married or not.

Does it hurt to have sex?

Sometimes sex does hurt, but kids don't need to know about sexual pain yet.

No, sex doesn't hurt. Sex can feel really good.

EXTRA INFO: Sometimes sex can hurt, but it usually doesn't.

What is an orgasm?

An orgasm is a really nice feeling that you can get during sex or when you touch your genitals in a nice way (masturbate).

What's an erection?

An erection is when your penis goes hard and erect.

EXTRA INFO: This happens because there is extra blood going into the penis.

EXTRA INFO: All males have erections, and they will start to have more of them as they get closer to puberty.

What does ejaculation mean?

Ejaculation is when semen, which contains sperm, comes out of the penis.

EXTRA INFO: The fluid comes out in little spurts, about a teaspoon in volume.

What is a virgin?

A virgin is someone who hasn't had sexual intercourse before.

How old do you have to be to have sex?

This answer depends on the law in the country and/or state that you live in. If you are unsure, just google 'legal age for sexual consent in (your state or country).'

The law says that you have to be (the legal age where you live). But in our family, we think that you shouldn't have sex until...' (you are married, in a loving and committed relationship, or whatever it is that you believe in).

Other sexual activities

Thanks to the oversexualised world we live in (and the porn that kids are exposed to), kids are hearing not just about baby-making-sex, but about all the other types of sex that can happen. Things like anal and oral sex, sexual fetishes, prostitution, bestiality, group sex, sex toys, B&D, S&M, pole dancing, stripping and more. So, you can find age-appropriate answers for questions about these things on page 122.

Masturbation

You will need to talk with your child about what your family values and beliefs are on masturbation. Try to talk about this in a way that will not leave your child feeling shame and guilt. Kids just see it as a part of their body that feels good when you touch it. We now see it as a normal sexual behaviour that is not harmful. You can learn more about how to talk in this article - https://sexedrescue.com/child-masturbation/

What is masturbation?

Masturbation is when you touch your penis or clitoris/vulva in a nice way and it feels good. People do it because it feels good.

EXTRA INFO: If a male is masturbating and their body has started to make sperm, they may ejaculate or come. This means that sticky white stuff called semen will come out of the end of their penis. There is usually a good feeling that goes with it called an orgasm.

Why do people masturbate?

Because it feels good.

EXTRA INFO: Usually because they have sexy feelings, i.e. tingly warm feelings in their body and genitals. Some people choose to masturbate when they have these feelings.

EXTRA INFO: Some people masturbate a lot, and some just sometimes. Some don't masturbate at all.

How do you masturbate with a penis?

They may rub or pull on the penis. If their body has started to make sperm, they will usually ejaculate and reach orgasm.

How do masturbate with a vulva?

They may touch or rub the vulva or clitoris. If they continue to rub and touch the clitoris and vulva, they might get a good feeling called an orgasm.

What is an orgasm?

An orgasm is a really nice feeling that you can get during sex or when you touch your genitals in a nice way (masturbate).

An orgasm is a really nice warm, tingly feeling around this area. It is a very strong feeling for a moment, and then it fades, leaving you with a warm, relaxed feeling.

Love, attraction and gender identity

You will find age-appropriate questions and answers about love and attraction and gender identity on page 108.

Contraception

Kids can understand that there are ways to stop a pregnancy from happening or continuing. They don't need to know about the details at this age as it really isn't relevant until they start thinking about sex as something that they might want to do.

What is contraception?

Contraception is something that you can do to prevent pregnancy.

EXTRA INFO: Contraception can be many different things. It could be a tablet that is taken each day, an injection every few months, an implant that goes into the arm or something that is inside the vagina or uterus.

If your religion doesn't believe in contraception, you will need to talk about natural methods instead. You could try saying, 'Our religion doesn't believe in contraception. So, to try to prevent pregnancy, we have sex when we are less likely to become pregnant.'

Can males use contraception?

Yes, they can. They can use something that will stop a female from becoming pregnant.

EXTRA INFO: Males can wear a condom to stop their sperm from going into the vagina. (A condom is like a special balloon that fits over the penis.)

EXTRA INFO: By the time you are an adult, there may even be an injection or a tablet that men can take. Some men can have a special operation that will stop their sperm from coming out (vasectomy).

What is a condom?

A condom is something that people use when they don't want to have babies.

EXTRA INFO: It is like a long, skinny balloon, and it covers the penis.

What is a vasectomy?

A special operation for males where the tube that carries the sperm from the testicles is cut and tied up so that no sperm can come out. Semen will still come out but there will be no sperm in it.

EXTRA INFO: The male will still make sperm but they will just get absorbed into their body, instead of coming out of the penis.

What is a tubal ligation?

A special operation for females where the tube that carries the egg is cut and tied so that the egg can't come out.

EXTRA INFO: The female will still release an egg each month but it will just get absorbed into their body.

What is an abortion?

An abortion (or termination) is when a person is pregnant and they can choose to have the pregnancy stopped.

EXTRA INFO: They might do this because there is something wrong with them or the baby or because they don't want to have a baby.

EXTRA INFO: They might have a special operation or take medicine that will make the pregnancy terminate (or finish).

If you are against terminating a pregnancy, you need to tell your child and explain why, e.g. 'I don't believe that people should have abortions because...'

Sexually Transmitted Infections (or STIs)

Kids will hear about STIs (sexually transmitted infections) and possibly even see the posters promoting screenings when using public bathrooms. They don't need to know all the details yet, as it isn't relevant. But it is important that they know that infections can be spread through sexual activity.

What is an STI?

If someone has germs or viruses in their vagina, penis or blood, they can pass the germs on to the person that they are having sex with. This means that the person that they are having sex with can get sick, too.

EXTRA INFO: Some STIs can last a lifetime. Most STIs are treatable, but some aren't.

EXTRA INFO: There are many different kinds of STIs. Some of them include genital warts, herpes, gonorrhoea, chlamydia, syphilis, HIV, hepatitis A, B and C, and pubic lice.

What is safe sex?

Safe sex means ways of having sex without getting any infections or becoming pregnant.

EXTRA INFO: It can mean a way to have sex where you don't get semen or vaginal fluid onto the other person's body.

EXTRA INFO: Condoms are one way of having safe sex.

What's AIDS?

AIDS is the name of a disease. It is caused by a virus called HIV (Human Immunodeficiency Virus).

EXTRA INFO: A virus is like a germ, in that it can make people get very sick.

EXTRA INFO: Sometimes you hear people talking about AIDS. When it first came out, a lot of people died from it, and because it was spread through sex and blood, a lot of people were scared.

How do people get AIDS?

They either need to have sexual intercourse with that person or share blood with them, like if you used someone else's drug needle after they had used it.

Penises, erections and wet dreams

Learn more about teaching your child the names of their genitals in this article – https://sexedrescue.com/naming-private-parts/. You can also find child-friendly diagrams to use with your child here - https://sexedrescue.com/products/.

Why is my friend's penis different?

Some penises are circumcised. This means that the skin on the end of their penis has been cut off. This means that the penis will look a little different at the end.

EXTRA INFO: Circumcision can happen for religious or cultural reasons, or because the foreskin can't stretch enough to be pushed back.

Why is my penis so small?

Penises come in all different sizes. Yours will grow bigger when you go through puberty. But for now, your penis is the right size for you.

What's an erection?

An erection is when your penis goes hard and erect.

EXTRA INFO: This happens when you have extra blood going into your penis.

EXTRA INFO: All males have erections and they will start to have more of them as they get closer to puberty.

EXTRA INFO: Erections are also an important part of making a baby. The penis has to be erect to let the sperm out. The penis also needs to be erect (or stiff) so that it can be pushed into the vagina.

Can I stop myself from having an erection?

During puberty, erections can happen for no reason at all. It can be very embarrassing for people when this happens.

EXTRA INFO: Unwanted erections will go away more quickly if you think of something else (like saying the alphabet backwards).

What is sperm?

Sperm is the male reproductive cell and is needed to make a baby.

What is semen?

Semen is the liquid that carries the sperm.

EXTRA INFO: Semen is sticky, cloudy (not clear) and whitish in colour.

EXTRA INFO: Its job is to keep the sperm healthy.

When will I start to make sperm?

Males usually start to make sperm when they are **13** and a half. Some will make it sooner and some will make it later.

What's a 'wet dream'?

A wet dream is when you ejaculate semen and sperm during your sleep. You might wake up when it happens, or you may just find a wet patch on your pants or sheets the next morning.

EXTRA INFO: Wet dreams only happen once your body starts to make semen and sperm.

EXTRA INFO: This is a normal thing to happen to males. Some males have many; some males, not as many; and some males never have a wet dream.

Can females have wet dreams?

Yes, they can have wet dreams too.

Puberty

Don't forget to remind your child that we all start puberty at different times. And that our bodies will all change differently. Breasts, penises and our bodies come in all different shapes and sizes. Reassure them that they are normal.

What is puberty?

Puberty is when your body changes from being a child to an adult body.

Why does puberty happen?

To get your body ready so that you can have a baby when you are all grown up.

What makes puberty happen?

Your body makes special chemicals called hormones. They make your body begin to change.

EXTRA INFO: The hormones are what make puberty happen. Hormones are chemicals that are made in different places throughout our bodies. Hormones travel through our bloodstream from the places that they are made to other places, which are where they make the changes.

The sex hormones are the hormones that make changes to the sex organs. For males, their testicles will make the hormone testosterone and sperm. For females, their ovaries will start producing progesterone and oestrogen, which then cause the egg (ovum or ova) to be released, breasts to grow, and periods to start. Other changes also start to happen throughout the body, like growing taller, pubic hair, etc.

How do the hormones get started?

When our body has grown to the right size and shape, it will trigger your brain to start sending messages to a small gland at the base of your brain called the pituitary gland, telling it to release growth hormones into your blood stream. The pituitary gland is 'the boss' hormone because it tells all the other glands what they need to do, to make puberty happen.

In males, the pituitary gland will tell your testicles to start producing sperm and the hormone testosterone.

In females, the pituitary gland will tell your ovaries to produce progesterone and oestrogen, which then causes the ova (eggs) to be released.

When will puberty happen?

Everybody is different. For most people it can be from as young as **8** or as late as **16**.

EXTRA INFO: Your body will start to change when it is the right size and shape for you.

EXTRA INFO: Females go through puberty first. Males usually start 2 years later.

What changes happen to female bodies?

- breasts begin to grow and develop
- hips become wider
- thighs and bottoms become more rounded
- armpit and pubic hair begin to grow
- body odour becomes stronger
- uterus, vagina and ovaries grow and begin to release eggs
- menstruation (periods) starts

What changes happen to male bodies?

- body shape becomes taller, heavier and more muscular, shoulders and chest broaden
- their voice begins to deepen

- armpit and pubic hair begin to grow
- body odour becomes stronger
- erections start happening more frequently (sometimes when you least expect them) and wet dreams occur more frequently
- penis, testicles and scrotum start to grow larger

How long will puberty last?

It is different for everyone, but it can be anytime between the ages of 8 and 18. It usually lasts for 4-5 years.

What happens when puberty is finished?

Nothing, you have now fully grown, i.e. an adult.

Why do some kids get embarrassed about puberty?

There are lots of reasons. Sometimes it can take a little bit of time to get used to, especially when other people can see the changes happening too. It can be pretty embarrassing for them when other people make comments about their new and different body.

They might be disappointed or sad that their childhood is finishing. Or scared about what it means to be an adult.

EXTRA INFO: Lots of kids feel embarrassed at some time during puberty

Why do we have to grow up?

It is something that just happens. You've already grown from being a helpless baby to a child who can do so much. Being an adult is just the next stage, and it has to happen so that you can reproduce and one day maybe have babies of your own.

Why do females start puberty first?

Females start puberty earlier because the pituitary gland is switched on earlier in them than it is in males.

How do I know when puberty is going to happen?

You won't really know until you start to see some changes in your own body. Everyone starts puberty at a different time. Some of your friends will start earlier, later or at the same time as you.

Why do your hormones go crazy during puberty?

The amount of hormones in your body can go up and down each day, which means that your emotions and feelings can go up and down too. Hormones make your body change physically but they also affect how you feel about your body and other people.

EXTRA INFO: Some days you may have high amounts and then other days you may have small amounts. This can sometimes make you feel a very different each day.

When will I start growing?

When your body is the right shape and size, your hormone body clock will start ticking. Which means that your body will start producing the sex hormones, which will make your body start to change.

Females can start growing from the ages of **8-9** and males usually start growing from around **11-12.**

When will I stop growing?

Females stop growing at around **16** years of age, and males at around **18.**

Why is my body so different than my friends'?

Everyone is different, which means that we all have different bodies. Some of us have blue eyes and some have brown eyes. Some of us have large breasts and some have small breasts. Either way, your body is special just the way it is.

EXTRA INFO: Puberty starts when your body is ready for it to start.

Why do I have man-boobs?

When puberty first starts, it is quite common for some males to have some swelling around their nipples, from the surge in hormones. It doesn't mean that they will be growing breasts. This swelling will settle down once their shoulders broaden and their muscles start to develop.

EXTRA INFO: It can take a few years for this to settle but don't worry, it is happening to other people too.

EXTRA INFO: Some people can also feel tender behind the nipple area. This will eventually go away as the hormone levels change.

When will I grow a beard?

Everyone is different, but usually sometime between the ages of 14 to 18. Facial hair is usually one of the last changes from puberty.

EXTRA INFO: When facial hair first starts to grow it usually looks like fluffy hair above the top lip and on your chin.

EXTRA INFO: How much hair you get depends on what the other men in your family have too.

Why does my voice sound different at times?

During puberty, your voice box (the larynx) is getting bigger. Because this growth happens very quickly, it can be hard for some people to control the pitch of their voice, especially if they are nervous. Their voice might sound squeaky or go up and down quickly.

This usually happens to males but it can happen to some females as well.

EXTRA INFO: This can be very embarrassing for most people.

When will I get pubic hair?

You'll get pubic hair anytime between the ages of 8 to 18. Everyone is different.

EXTRA INFO: Most people start to notice it from between 11-14 years old.

Why is my pubic hair changing and getting curly?

That is perfectly normal and is just something that happens as you get more and more pubic hair.

Is pubic hair straight or curly?

Pubic hair can be straight or curly and it depends on your cultural background. It can also feel a bit coarser (or rougher) than the hair on your head.

EXTRA INFO: The type of pubic hair that you have is inherited from your family.

Is your pubic hair the same colour as the hair on your head?

It usually is, but not always.

EXTRA INFO: Blonde people usually have darker pubic hair.

How hairy will I get?

That depends, as it is different for everyone. Some cultural backgrounds have more hair than others.

EXTRA INFO: There are ways to get rid of body hair if you don't want it but we can talk about that when it happens.

Why do some females get fat at puberty?

They don't necessarily get fatter, but their bodies do begin to change in anticipation of one day having a baby. Their hips will get wider, which means that there is room for their uterus to grow during pregnancy.

Do some females never get their periods?

Some people don't get their period, but that isn't very common. If they don't have their period by the time they are **16**, they usually go and see a doctor about this.

When will my breasts stop growing?

They will usually stop growing by the end of puberty when you are around **18**.

EXTRA INFO: Because breasts are made of fatty tissue, they can grow larger if you increase your body weight.

Why is one of my breasts bigger than the other?

Sometimes this is just what happens. They usually catch up with each other by the time you have finished growing. Most people don't have perfectly matched breasts.

EXTRA INFO: This is happening to other people too, but no one else will notice but you!

Why do I get white stuff on my underpants?

That is something that happens to your body as you start puberty. We call it vaginal discharge and it is the vagina's way of cleaning itself.

Why do I sometimes feel wet in my vagina/vulva area?

That is a slippery liquid called mucous. It is supposed to be there and it keeps your vagina and cervix moist.

EXTRA INFO: Your mucous will change in colour and texture because of the hormones during your menstrual cycle. When an egg is released from the ovary, the mucous is usually slippery and clear like egg white, which helps the sperm to travel more quickly to the egg. At other times of the month, it can be whiter, and even yellowish too.

How big will my vulva grow?

Just like we have different sized feet, we can have differently sized and shaped vulvas. They come in all different sizes, shapes and colours, but you usually end up with the right size vulva for your body.

What's menopause?

Menopause is when the female body stops being fertile. It means that you can no longer naturally conceive and grow a baby.

EXTRA INFO: The ovaries will stop releasing eggs and uterus will stop making the thick lining that is needed to receive the fertilised eggs.

What's ovulation?

Ovulation is when the ovary releases a mature egg into the fallopian tubes, ready to be fertilised.

Do you feel the egg being released?

Not usually, but some people do. They might feel a twinge in their tummy area that doesn't last long.

Periods

If you are female, you will be able to answer most of these questions by yourself! As you've got lots of personal experience with periods already!

If your child has a uterus, you will want to have a 'period kit' made up, that they can keep in their school bag. You can read more about how to make one up - https://sexedrescue.com/diy-period-kit-for-school/. And you can learn about the different menstrual products here - http://sexedrescue.com/menstruation-products/.

Don't forget to remind your child that we all start puberty at different times. And that our bodies will all change differently. Breasts, penises and our bodies come in all different shapes and sizes. Reassure them that they are normal.

What's a period?

A period is a small amount of blood that comes out of a vagina every month.

EXTRA INFO: Each month the body prepares itself in case a baby is made. The uterus makes a special lining which is ready for the fertilised egg to land on, which is where it will then grow into a baby. If a baby doesn't happen, the lining is no longer needed. The lining then comes out through the vagina as menstrual blood or a period. Your body will do this each month.

EXTRA INFO: This cycle will keep on happening until your hormones tell it to stop.

What's the menstrual cycle?

The amount of time between the first day of your period and the day before your next period starts. So, if a person got their period on January 1 and then again on January 29, their cycle will have lasted 28 days.

The menstrual cycle is the changes that your body goes through every month to prepare for pregnancy.

EXTRA INFO: When you first start your periods, your cycle can be anywhere between 21-45 days. After a few years, it will decrease to 21-36 days. Everyone is different.

Can males have periods?

Some children will have the reproductive organs of a female but feel like a boy on the inside. They will have periods until they begin transitioning to become a boy.

Not usually, because you need a uterus to have a period, and it is usually females who have a uterus.

How many days do you bleed for?

A period usually lasts between 3 to 7 days, and it usually happens each month.

EXTRA INFO: Only a small amount of blood comes out – about a third of a cup.

Why do people have periods?

It is a part of the what the body does, to get ready for falling pregnant. Each month the uterus makes a special lining of blood to grow a baby onto. When a baby isn't made, the special lining isn't needed, so it comes out of the vagina as blood.

When do you stop getting your period?

Your period can stop if you are pregnant. It can also stop because of stress, illness, changes in your body weight and even a change in routine, like going on holiday!

EXTRA INFO: Eventually your period will stop when you are about 50 and reach menopause.

EXTRA INFO: Menopause is when your body stops being fertile. It means that you can no longer naturally conceive and grow a baby.

How will you know when you get your period?

You will feel some wetness around your vagina and find a small amount of blood on your undies or when you wipe after going to the toilet.

EXTRA INFO: The blood will change colour from day to day, from pink to red to brown.

EXTRA INFO: Some people get moody around the time of their period.

How often will I get my period?

Periods happen every **3** to **6** weeks.

EXTRA INFO: The average time is 28 days, but it can vary from between 21-36 days. The timing of your period can be affected by things like stress, illness, changes in your body weight and even a change in routine, like going on holiday!

EXTRA INFO: During puberty, periods are not very regular and the average length of time that they last is between 2-8 days.

When will I get my period?

Some people can be as young as **8** or as old as **16** before they start their period.

Can you get your period when you are pregnant?

No, you can't. Your body will know that it is pregnant and that the lining of the uterus is needed.

Do you sometimes wake up in puddles of blood, when you have your period?

You won't wake up in a puddle of blood, but you might leak blood during the night, staining your pyjamas and or sheets.

EXTRA INFO: You can use a heavier pad during the night, that will hold more blood.

Does it hurt when you have your period?

Some people might get a twinge in the pelvic area, but most people keep on doing whatever they are normally doing.

Some people can get cramping in the pelvic area or a lower back ache that gets better after a day or two. Some will take pain relief or use a hot pack to help relax the muscles in the pelvic area or lower back.

EXTRA INFO: Eventually your period becomes more regular and predictable once puberty has finished.

How can I keep track of when my period is due?

You can track of when they started in a diary or even download an app to your phone/tablet. This way you can try to work out what your pattern is, and you will have a good idea of when your period is likely to arrive.

When will my periods become regular?

It can take between 2 to 3 years for your periods to become regular.

How much blood do you lose during your period?

About a third to one-half of a cup of blood. It might seem like a lot more than that!

EXTRA INFO: Everyone is different. Some lose more blood, or less blood, than others.

Why do I get cramps during my period?

Your uterus contracts (tightens and relaxes). This helps to remove the lining from the walls of your uterus, which then comes our as menstrual blood.

EXTRA INFO: Some people get more cramping than others.

Can you swim when you have your period?

You can, but you will need to use a tampon or swimpants. You can't swim with a pad because it will swell up from the water, may even start to fall apart and it will be pretty easy for everyone to know that you are wearing a pad. If you swim without a tampon, the blood will be diluted but it will still run down your leg, which means that people will see it. So, most people choose to not go swimming when they have their period (unless they are using tampons or swimpants).

What's PMS?

Some people experience a range of different emotional and physical symptoms for a week or so before they get their period, and sometimes even during their period.

Symptoms can include: cramps, backaches, breast tenderness, skin problems, bloating, mild depression, headaches, and/or angry outbursts.

EXTRA INFO: Everyone is different so you may or may not get some of these symptoms. Plus, there are things that we can do to help make you feel better, if you do get any of them.

What do you need for a period?

When you first start, you will be using pads. They have a sticky strip and will stick to the inside of your underpants.

EXTRA INFO: When you are a little bit older, you can look at using tampons. They are inserted into your vagina and absorb the blood inside there.

What are pads?

A pad is something that you use to absorb blood when you have your period. You wear it in your underpants and it sits between your legs, touching your vulva.

EXTRA INFO: It has a sticky strip that helps it to attach to your underpants and to stay there in place.

Why do some pads have wings?

Some pads do have wings. They wrap around the crotch of your underpants and can help to stop the blood from going onto them. Some wings have an absorbent material and will stop the pad from leaking in the middle.

How often do you need to change your pad?

When the pad looks full towards the centre, it is usually a good time to change it. Every 3-4 hours is a good frequency, which means during recess and lunch breaks whilst at school. You can sleep in the one pad at night, and just change it when you wake up.

EXTRA INFO: If the pad feels wet or soggy, it means that it needs to be changed.

EXTRA INFO: Pads can start to smell after about 5-6 hours, especially on a hot and sweaty day.

How long do pads last?

A pad will last anywhere between 2 to 7 hours, depending on your blood flow. If you are bleeding more heavily, the pad won't last as long.

Why are there so many different types of pads?

It can get pretty confusing when you look at all the different types of pads. Basically, some are just longer or shorter, wider or narrower, thicker or thinner, heavier or lighter. The companies that make them have come up with lots of different fancy names.

Can I flush pads down the toilet?

No, there is a good chance that it will block the toilet. If there isn't a bin in the toilet cubicle, you can wrap the pad up into the packet that the new pad came out of (or in lots of toilet paper) and place it in the bin next to the hand basin.

EXTRA INFO: Some people have a special period kit that they take to the toilet with them. You can keep plastics bags in there that are for holding used pads and tampons. You can use this to hold any used pads, and just throw them away when you get home.

What are panty liners for?

Panty liners are a much smaller, thinner pad that will hold a small amount of blood or vaginal discharge.

What is a tampon?

A tampon is something that you insert into your vagina to catch the blood before it comes out. It is a finger-shaped wad of absorbent material, just like what is in pads.

EXTRA INFO: Vaginas are very stretchy and have no trouble holding a tampon.

Do I have to use tampons?

No, only if you want to. Most people start off with using pads and then start using tampons because they want to play sport whilst they have their period.

EXTRA INFO: Everyone is different. Some people don't use tampons, some people use both tampons and pads, and some people only use tampons.

How do I put a tampon in?

Some people are fine with using tampons but some are more nervous. If they can insert a finger fully into their vagina, they should be fine with inserting a tampon. Sometimes it can help if they use a dab of vaginal lubricant on the tip of the tampon. This helps the tampon to glide in rather than drag in. You can also buy small tampons or tampons that are covered in a silky covering that make insertion much easier.

They aren't that hard to put in. Inside the tampon packet, you will find some instructions on how to insert them. First, you find a position that is comfortable. You can squat, sit down on the toilet or stand with leg up on the toilet. You take the tampon out of its wrapper, part the opening to your vagina, and push the tampon up into your vagina.

We can talk about this more when you are ready to start using tampons.

Do tampons hurt when you insert them?

Some people may want to practice inserting a tampon before they have their next period. This will be uncomfortable and difficult to do. So, make sure that they know that they know that they need to actually be bleeding, and the heavier their flow, the easier it will be to insert that first tampon.

If you try to insert a tampon into a vagina that isn't bleeding, it will be uncomfortable.

It won't hurt but it can be uncomfortable. If you can relax, it means that the muscles around the vagina will soften and loosen, which means that it will be easier to push the tampon in. You do have to make sure, though, that you are bleeding at the time.

EXTRA INFO: It is a good idea to wait until you have had your period for a few years before you start using tampons. By then your vagina will have finished growing, and it will be easier to insert the tampon.

EXTRA INFO: Sometimes you can put a dab of lubricant on the end of the tampon to make it easier for it to go in. This has to be proper vagina lubricant and should be freshly opened (not opened up years ago).

How do I know where to put the tampon?

Some people are totally ignorant of what they have below. So, they may need some encouragement to go and grab a mirror and to have a look at what they actually have between their legs.

The tampon goes into the vagina, the middle opening. There is only one opening that is big enough for a tampon. It is the one that you can feel if you have a little feel in your vulva area.

How long do I leave the tampon in for?

It all depends on how heavy your blood flow is, but it could need changing as often as every **2-6** hours. Your confidence with using tampons will increase, as you start using them.

EXTRA INFO: It is harder to tell when a tampon is full, as the blood is all inside. When it is getting full, the tampon string will be stained with blood and blood will leak onto your underpants. Some people like to wear a small pad or panty liner until they are more confident with using tampons.

Can I use a tampon overnight?

You shouldn't use a tampon overnight as they need to be changed every **6-8** hours. Plus, it could be unsafe because of Toxic Shock Syndrome (TSS).

EXTRA INFO: Toxic Shock Syndrome (TSS) is a rare bacterial infection that is linked to the use of tampons. It is rare but can kill women.

How do I get the tampon out?

There is a string at the end of the tampon that stays outside the vagina when you insert it. When you tug at the string, the tampon will slide out.

Can a tampon fall out?

No, once it is in the vagina, it will stay there. If you haven't pushed it up far enough into the vagina, it might feel uncomfortable though.

What happens if a tampon gets stuck up there?

It is pretty uncommon for a tampon to get stuck. Sometimes, though, they can be a bit tricky to remove, usually because there is not enough moisture in them.

If one does get stuck, you can try squatting down and relaxing the vaginal muscles as you pull down. You can also try putting clean fingers into the vagina to help pull the tampon out. If it gets too stressful, stop for half an hour and then go back and try again.

EXTRA INFO: If it does get stuck, you can ring your local Women's Health Centre, STI Clinic or doctor for it to be removed. Make sure you tell them when you call so that you get an appointment that day.

Can I flush tampons down the toilet?

No, there is a good chance that it will block the toilet. If there isn't a bin in the toilet cubicle, you can wrap the tampon up in lots of paper and place it in the bins next to the hand basin.

EXTRA INFO: Some people have a special period kit that they take to the toilet with them. You can keep plastics bags in there that are for holding used pads and tampons. You can use this to hold any used tampons, and just throw them away when you get home.

Can you still go to the toilet if you have a tampon in?

Yes, you can. Your urine will just run out as it normally does. You may want to lift the tampon string out of the way though so that it doesn't get wet!

Are tampons dangerous?

Tampons aren't dangerous if they are used properly. You need to have clean hands, and not leave them in the vagina for too long. Tampons have been linked with a rare but serious infection called Toxic Shock Syndrome (TSS).

You can access my FREE sex education course for parents at https://sexedrescue.com/back-to-basics/

12 YEAR OLDS

Babies (and how they are made)

> Try to get into the habit of explaining what you think or believe when talking about love, sex and relationships. This is your opportunity to guide your child as they grow up, and to help them make healthy decisions around love, sex and relationships.

How are babies made?

> If your child wants a technical explanation, it can get complicated. The best way to explain this is to watch this simple video from the Khan Academy together: https://www.khanacademy.org/test-prep/mcat/cells/embryology/v/egg-sperm-and-fertilization

A baby is made (or conceived) when sperm from the male joins with an egg/ovum from the female.

This usually happens when the male ejaculates semen (which contains sperm) into the vagina. The sperm then travel up through the cervix (which is the opening of the uterus), into the uterus and then into the fallopian tubes, looking for an egg to fertilize. If the sperm joins with an egg, a baby is formed.

EXTRA INFO: You need a cell from a male and a female, as it needs both parts to join for a baby to be made. A female cannot make a baby without sperm, and a male cannot make a baby without an ovum or egg.

EXTRA INFO: Some animals can reproduce without requiring a cell from another animal. This is called parthenogenesis. Humans, though, need cells from both a male and a female to reproduce.

What other ways can a baby be made?

Babies can also be made in other ways. IVF, or in vitro fertilization, is a medical procedure where the sperm and eggs are joined together outside the uterus. Egg or sperm donation is where someone gives you an egg or sperm to use. Surrogacy is where a person will become pregnant and grow a baby for someone else. There is also adoption, where a person will give away a baby that they cannot care for.

How do you get twins?

Twins happen in 2 different ways. Identical twins will happen when a single egg splits into two after it has been fertilized. Identical twins share the same genes, are the same sex and look almost the same.

Non-identical, or fraternal, twins will happen when 2 eggs leave the ovaries at the same time, and each egg is fertilized by a separate sperm. These twins do not share the same genes, may not be the same sex and may not look the same.

How is the egg made into a baby?

Once the sperm joins with the egg, it begins to divide into even more cells. This creates something called DNA, which is like a set of instructions on how the baby should grow.

How long does it take for the sperm to find the egg?

Anywhere from half an hour to 5 days.

How does the sperm know where to go?

There is a chemical in the fluid around the egg that attracts the sperm. The female also has special mucus in their vagina and cervix that helps the sperm to travel into the uterus.

Do you have to have sex every time you want a baby?

Yes, you do. Unless you have trouble becoming pregnant or you don't have a partner, and then you can seek medical assistance to get pregnant.

How many times do you need to have sex to make a baby?

You only need to have sex once to make a baby, but sometimes it takes more than one attempt to make a baby.

Can you make a baby every time you have sex?

No, you can't make a baby every time. The female is only fertile for a few days of each month. So, timing to make a baby is pretty important.

What happens to the sperm if there is no egg?

The sperm will eventually run out of energy and die. They are so small that they are then just absorbed into the female's body. If this happens, no baby is made.

How do you get a male or female baby?

This can get complicated. The best way to explain this is to watch this simple video from the Khan Academy: https://www.khanacademy.org/test-prep/mcat/cells/embryology/v/egg-sperm-and-fertilization

The sex of the baby is determined by the sperm. Eggs carry an X chromosome, whereas sperm will carry an X and Y chromosome.

If an egg is fertilized by a sperm with a Y chromosome, it will make a male baby (X + Y = male). If the egg is fertilized by a sperm with the X chromosome, it will make a female baby (X + X = female).

What are genes?

Your genes are the instructions that work out how you will be made. They determine if you will be a male or a female, have green or blue eyes, or have red or brown hair, etc. Your genes are passed down to you from your parents, and through them from their parents, and so on.

EXTRA INFO: Your genes are made up of DNA, or Deoxyribonucleic acid, which carries your genes.

How old do you have to be to have a baby?

Males need to be making sperm before they can help to make a baby. So that could be anytime from the age of **13** or **14**.

Females need to be having their periods before they can become pregnant. So that could be anytime from the age of **10-11**.

You can also add a value statement about when you feel they should be having babies, e.g. 'In our family, we believe that you shouldn't have sex until...' (you are married, in a loving and committed relationship, are 16 or whatever it is that you believe in).

Sexual intercourse

Your child will have already heard about sex at the playground, from their friends and through the media. This means that you have to be prepared for questions about sexual activities that are not age-appropriate, like bestiality (having sex with animals). Answering their questions will satisfy their curiosity and allow them to move on to something else, like, 'What's for dinner?' If you don't satisfy their curiosity, they may just go looking for an answer elsewhere, e.g. their friends or the internet.

If your child starts to ask questions about the different types of sexual behavior, it is usually a good idea to find out why they are asking the question. You could very casually say, 'Why are you asking that?' or, 'Where did you hear that word?'

You can add a value statement about the situations in which you believe sex should happen, e.g. 'In our family, we believe that you shouldn't have sex until...' (you are married, in a loving and committed relationship, are 16, or whatever it is that you believe in).

What is sex?

At first, kids are only curious about sex because they want to know how babies are made or they have heard whispers and giggles about this thing called sex. So, when we first start talking about sex (sexual intercourse), we can just talk about baby-making sex, i.e. sexual intercourse. Later on, we start adding in that there is a bit more to sex like hugging, kissing, etc. And that adults also have sex for other reasons as well. And we always remind kids that sex is something that adults do and that it is not for kids.

Sex can be lots of different things, but usually, when you hear people talking about sex, they are talking about sexual intercourse, i.e. penis in vagina sex.

When two adults like each other a lot, they may want to have sexual intercourse with each other. This means that they may hug, kiss and touch each other's bodies all over. The penis becomes erect and the vagina becomes moist and slippery. This makes it easier for the penis to go into the vagina. The male pushes their penis into the vagina (or the female lets the male push their penis into the vagina), they hold each other close, they move around a bit and it can feel good. After a while, the male almost always ejaculates.

EXTRA INFO: Adults have sexual intercourse because they like the way it feels. Their whole body feels good, not just their genitals.

EXTRA INFO: Sexual intercourse is something very private and should happen with (insert your values).

What is casual sex?

Casual sex with someone that you don't know or aren't in a relationship with is more common nowadays. So, make sure you talk about the fact that it does happen, and talk about how you feel about it. Try to have a conversation with your child and talk about what they think, too.

EXTRA INFO: Some people have sex with someone that they don't know very well. It could be a complete stranger, or someone that they have met before.

What is foreplay?

Foreplay is the name for all the other stuff, like cuddling and kissing and touching each other's bodies. The stuff that helps to get you into the mood for sex.

What happens when you have sex?

Eventually your child will realize that adults don't just have sex to make babies. So, you can also start talking about how adults often kiss, hug, touch and engage in other sexual behaviors with one another to show caring for each other and to feel good.

There are lots of different ways to have sex. The main way that adults have sex to make a baby is when the penis goes vagina. They also do other things like hug, kiss, and touch each other's bodies in a nice way.

EXTRA INFO: Sex is something that most people do when they are grown up.

How do two females have sex?

You don't need to go into great detail here. Keep it simple!

There is more to sex than penises and vaginas. It is also about kissing, hugging, and touching each other's genitals. Gay (or lesbian) females can do all of this except for putting a penis in a vagina.

How do two males have sex?

You don't need to go into great detail here. Keep it simple!

There is more to sex than penises and vaginas. It is also about kissing, hugging, and touching each other's genitals. Gay males can do all of this except for putting a penis in a vagina.

Will I ever want to have sex?

Some kids will experience stronger or weaker sexual feelings than others. Some kids will start to have sexual feelings sooner or later than other kids. Everyone is different.

You probably will one day. During puberty, you will start to think about sex differently. This is because of your hormones.

EXTRA INFO: You might find that you start thinking about someone in a new way. You may think about them a lot, have butterflies in your stomach when you meet and daydream about holding hands with them, hugging and kissing.

Will I have sex one day?

Yes, you probably will have sex one day, but it won't be until you are an adult.

You can also add a value statement about when you think they can have sex, e.g. 'In our family, we believe that you shouldn't have sex until...' (you are married, in a loving and committed relationship, or whatever it is that you believe in).

When will I want to have sex?

Kids sometimes struggle to understand why they might ever want to have sex one day. One way to explain this is to talk about our 'sex switch.' That switch doesn't get turned on until puberty. Once the switch is turned on, it slowly starts to rewire your brain so that you see sex as something that you want to do instead of something that is weird or gross.

You won't be interested in having sex until puberty happens. Once your body starts making hormones, you will start to think about sex and people in a different way.

EXTRA INFO: Most people don't just have sex with a complete stranger. They usually start off by getting to know another person first, then become friends. The couple will usually hold hands, hug, cuddle and kiss before they get to the sex part.

Why do people have sex?

Adults have sex for lots of different reasons. To make babies, to show their love for each other, for fun, because it feels good, or to make you feel closer to each other. Having sex is a natural, normal and healthy part of life.

EXTRA INFO: Having sex with someone can be a very intimate experience to share. You can connect with your partner at the most intimate and knowing level that there is.

EXTRA INFO: A lot of things usually happen before a relationship becomes sexual. The two people usually start off being friends first and will hold hands, hug, cuddle and kiss before they get to the sex part.

Where do adults have sex?

Usually somewhere private, like in their bedroom.

EXTRA INFO: Sex is a private activity.

Do you have to lie down to have sex?

If you want to, you can. There are lots of different ways that adults can position their bodies to have sexual intercourse.

Do you have to be married to have sex?

The answer to this question depends on your personal beliefs.

Yes, in our family/church we believe that you need to be married to have sex.

OR

No, in our family we don't believe that you need to be married first. But we believe that you need to be an adult and in a loving and committed relationship first (or say what you believe in).

EXTRA INFO: But, physically, your grownup body is capable of having sex whether you are married or not.

Does it hurt to have sex?

Sometimes sex does hurt, but kids don't need to know about sexual pain yet.

Sex doesn't usually hurt. Sex can feel really good.

EXTRA INFO: Sometimes sex can hurt, but it usually doesn't.

What's a lubricant?

Lubricant is something that your body makes naturally so that it is easier for the penis to go into the vagina (or anus).

EXTRA INFO: You can also buy lubricant as a gel or liquid, in a tube or bottle, that you can use as well.

What is an orgasm?

An orgasm is a really nice feeling that you can get during sex or when you touch your genitals in a nice way (masturbate). For males, it usually happens when the semen comes out of the penis. For females, it can happen when the outside of the vulva and/or clitoris is rubbed or during vaginal penetration.

An orgasm usually happens when pleasure builds up through sexual intercourse or masturbation. So, you have to be sexually excited and turned on for an orgasm to happen.

Orgasms feel really, really good and are one of the many good things about sex.

EXTRA INFO: Orgasms don't happen every time you have sexual activity. You can still enjoy sex without an orgasm.

EXTRA INFO: Our bodies want us to reproduce, so nature has helped by making sure that sex can feel really good. An orgasm is one of these good things.

How do you have an orgasm?

Orgasms can happen during sexual intercourse, masturbation and when a male has a wet dream. They don't just happen randomly. They happen because of sexual pleasure.

What's an erection?

An erection is when the penis goes hard and erect.

EXTRA INFO: This happens when there is extra blood going into the penis.

EXTRA INFO: All males have erections, and they will start to have more of them as they get closer to puberty.

What does ejaculation mean?

Ejaculation is when semen, which contains sperm, comes out of the penis.

EXTRA INFO: The fluid comes out in little spurts, about a teaspoon in volume.

What is a virgin?

A virgin is someone who hasn't had sexual intercourse before.

How old do you have to be to have sex?

This answer depends on the law in the country and/or state that you live in. If you are unsure, just google 'legal age for sexual consent in (your state or country).'

The law says that you have to be (the legal age where you live). But in our family, we think that you shouldn't have sex until...' (you are married, in a loving and committed relationship, or whatever it is that you believe in).

Other sexual activities

Thanks to the oversexualised world we live in (and the porn that kids are exposed to), kids are hearing not just about baby-making-sex, but about all the other types of sex that can happen. Things like anal and oral sex, sexual fetishes, prostitution, bestiality, group sex, sex toys, B&D, S&M, pole dancing, stripping and more. So, you can find age-appropriate answers for questions about these things on page 122.

Masturbation

You will need to talk with your child about what your family values and beliefs are on masturbation. Try to talk about this in a way that will not leave your child feeling shame and guilt. Kids just see it as a part of their body that feels good when you touch it. We now see it as a normal sexual behaviour that is not harmful. You can learn more about how to talk in this article - https://sexedrescue.com/child-masturbation/

What is masturbation?

Masturbation is when you touch your penis or clitoris/vulva in a nice way and it feels good. People do it because it feels good.

EXTRA INFO: If a male is masturbating and their body has started to make sperm, they may ejaculate or come. This means that sticky white stuff called semen will come out of the end of their penis. There is usually a good feeling that goes with it called an orgasm.

Why do people masturbate?

People masturbate for lots of reasons but they usually do it because it feels good. Masturbation usually ends up with an orgasm, which is a really nice feeling that you get when you are sexually excited (or aroused).

EXTRA INFO: Some people masturbate a lot, and some just sometimes. Some don't masturbate at all.

Is it normal to masturbate?

Yes, it is normal to masturbate and is a way that kids can get to know how their bodies feel and work.

EXTRA INFO: Some people masturbate more than others. Some people don't masturbate at all. Everyone is different and that is okay.

EXTRA INFO: The hormones during puberty can create lots of sexy feelings, which make kids want to masturbate more.

Is it wrong to masturbate?

There is no research that proves that masturbation is harmful.

EXTRA INFO: Some religions and cultures, though, believe that masturbation is wrong.

EXTRA INFO: Too much masturbation can be a problem. If it is something that you have to do, and if it stops you from doing other things, it can be a problem.

EXTRA INFO: Some kids watch porn to masturbate. This isn't a good thing to do because it may cause problems for you when you are older and in a sexual relationship with someone.

You will need to talk with your child about what your family values and beliefs are on masturbation. Try to talk about this in a way that will not leave your child feeling shame and guilt.

How do you masturbate with a penis?

They may rub or pull on the penis. If their body has started to make sperm, they will usually ejaculate and reach orgasm.

How do masturbate with a vulva?

They may touch or rub the vulva or clitoris. If they continue to rub and touch the clitoris and vulva, they might get a good feeling called an orgasm.

What is an orgasm?

An orgasm is a really nice feeling that you can get during sex or when you touch your genitals in a nice way (masturbate).

EXTRA INFO: An orgasm is a really nice warm, tingly feeling around this area. It is a very strong feeling for a moment, and then it fades, leaving you with a warm, relaxed feeling.

Why do orgasms happen?

Orgasm usually happen with pleasure built up through sexual intercourse or masturbation. So, you have to be sexually excited and turned on for an orgasm to happen.

Orgasms feel really, really good and are one of the many good things about sex.

EXTRA INFO: Orgasms don't happen every time you have sexual activity. You can still enjoy sex without an orgasm.

EXTRA INFO: Our bodies want us to reproduce, so nature has helped by making sure that sex can feel really good. Orgasm is one of these good things.

How do you have an orgasm?

Orgasm can happen during sexual intercourse, masturbation and when a male has a wet dream.

Love, attraction and gender identity

You will find age-appropriate questions and answers about love and attraction and gender identity on page 108.

Contraception

12-year-olds can understand that there are ways to stop a pregnancy from happening or continuing. They don't need to know all the details yet, as it isn't relevant. But it is important that they know that adults can choose whether or not to have a baby.

What is abstinence?

Abstinence is when a person decides to not have sexual intercourse.

What is contraception?

Contraception is something that you can do to prevent pregnancy.

EXTRA INFO: Contraception can be many different things. It could be a tablet that is taken each day, an injection every few months, an implant that goes into the arm or something that is inside the vagina or uterus. Or you can even have surgery.

If your religion doesn't believe in contraception, you will need to talk about natural methods instead. You could try saying, 'Our religion doesn't believe in contraception. So, to try to prevent pregnancy, we have sex when we are less likely to become pregnant.'

Can males use contraception?

Yes, they can. They can use something that will stop a female from becoming pregnant.

EXTRA INFO: Males can wear a condom to stop their sperm from going into the vagina. (A condom is like a special balloon that fits over the penis.)

EXTRA INFO: By the time you are an adult, there may even be an injection or a tablet that men can take. Some males can have a special operation that will stop their sperm from coming out (vasectomy).

What is a condom?

A condom is like a long, skinny balloon, and it covers the penis. It catches the sperm and stops it from going into the other person's body.

What is a vasectomy?

A special operation for males where the tube that carries the sperm from the testicles is cut and tied up so that no sperm can come out. Semen will still come out, but there will be no sperm in it.

EXTRA INFO: The male will still make sperm but they will just get absorbed into their body, instead of coming out of the penis.

What is a tubal ligation?

A special operation for females where the tube that carries the egg is cut and tied so that the egg can't come out.

EXTRA INFO: The female will still release an egg each month but it will just get absorbed into their body.

What is an abortion?

An abortion (or termination) is when a person is pregnant and they can choose to have the pregnancy stopped.

EXTRA INFO: They might do this because there is something wrong with them or the baby or because they don't want to have a baby.

EXTRA INFO: They might have a special operation or take medicine that will make the pregnancy terminate (or finish).

If you are against terminating a pregnancy, you need to tell your child and explain why, e.g. 'I don't believe that people should have abortions because...'

Sexually Transmitted Infections (or STIs)

STIs (sexually transmitted infections) is the current term that we use to describe the things that you can catch when having sex.

When talking about STIs, make sure that you also talk about your family values and religious beliefs in regards to when it is okay for your child to start having sex. It is important to keep on talking about what sexual behaviors and attitudes are okay and not okay in your family, so that your child knows what is expected.

What is an STI?

If someone has germs or viruses in their vagina, penis or blood, they can pass the germs on to the person that they are having sex with. This means that the person that they are having sex with can get sick, too.

EXTRA INFO: Some STIs can last a lifetime. Most STIs are treatable, but some aren't.

What is safe sex?

Safe sex means ways of having sex without getting any infections or becoming pregnant.

EXTRA INFO: It can mean a way to have sex where you don't get semen or vaginal fluid onto the other person's body.

EXTRA INFO: Condoms are one way of having safe sex.

What are the different types of STIs?

These are the most common STIs. There are other ones as well that are not as common.

There are many different types of STIs. Some are easier to catch than others. Some can be treated, while others can last a lifetime. Some are more common than others.

There are bacterial STIs, like chlamydia, gonorrhoea, and syphilis. These can be treated, but can sometimes cause long-term damage if left untreated.

There are viral STIs, like genital warts, genital herpes, hepatitis and HIV/AIDS. There is no treatment that will get rid of these viruses, but the symptoms can be treated.

Then there are the parasitic STIs, like scabies and crabs. These can be treated with skin washes and shampoos.

How will I know if I have an STI?

You might have a discharge from your vagina or penis, or find sores, redness, a rash or irritation in the genital area; it might hurt to have sex, or burn when you pass urine.

EXTRA INFO: Sometimes you may not know that you have an STI. This means that you can infect other people without even knowing.

How do you prevent STIs?

You might use a condom, which will stop any infections from getting inside your penis or vagina. A condom will prevent most STIs, but not all.

EXTRA INFO: Once you start having sex, you can also start having STI checks, which is where they test you for any infections that you may have caught through sexual contact.

What's unprotected sex?

Unprotected sex means having vaginal, anal or oral sex without using a condom. Which means that you are at risk of STIs and possibly even pregnancy if you haven't used any contraception.

What's AIDS?

AIDS is the name of a disease. It is caused by a virus called HIV (Human Immunodeficiency Virus).

EXTRA INFO: A virus is like a germ, in that it can make people get very sick.

EXTRA INFO: Sometimes you hear people talking about AIDS. When it first came out, a lot of people died from it, and because it was spread through sex and blood, a lot of people were scared.

How do people get AIDS?

They either need to have sexual intercourse with that person or share blood with them, like if you used someone else's drug needle after they had used it.

Penises and erections

Don't forget to remind your child that we all start puberty at different times. And that our bodies will all change differently. Breasts, penises and our bodies come in all different shapes and sizes. Reassure them that they are normal.

You can also find child-friendly diagrams to use with your child here - https://sexedrescue.com/products/

Why is my friend's penis different?

Some penises are circumcised. This means that the skin on the end of their penis has been cut off. This means that the penis will look a little different at the end.

EXTRA INFO: Circumcision can happen for religious or cultural reasons, or because the foreskin can't stretch enough to be pushed back.

Why is my penis so small?

Penises come in all different sizes. Yours will grow bigger when you go through puberty. But for now, your penis is the right size for you.

What is an erection?

An erection is when the amount of blood going to the penis increases, making the penis hard and erect.

EXTRA INFO: An erect penis is much bigger than a soft one and stands away from the body.

EXTRA INFO: All males have erections but during puberty, they happen more often.

EXTRA INFO: Sometimes erections happen for no reason at all. You don't have to be sexually aroused to have an erection.

Why do I have erections?

All males have erections, and even little kids and babies get them too.

They can happen when you are having sexy thoughts when the penis is touched or rubbed by clothing. Sometimes they can happen for no reason at all.

Can I stop myself from having an erection?

During puberty, erections can happen for no reason at all. It can be very embarrassing for people when this happens.

EXTRA INFO: Unwanted erections will go away more quickly if you think of something else (like saying the alphabet backwards).

EXTRA INFO: Unwanted erections won't happen forever. Once puberty is over, you will find that you have more control over your erections.

Why do I wake up with an erection?

It is common for people to wake up with an erection. They usually happen during the REM (Rapid Eye Movement) phase of sleep, which is just before you wake up. Sometimes it can also be because you have a full bladder.

EXTRA INFO: If you happen to have a sexy dream during this phase, you will sometimes ejaculate.

EXTRA INFO: A full bladder can place pressure on the erectile tissue at the base of the penis, causing an erection. Because you can't wee with an erection, you will have to wait a few minutes for your penis to relax before you can pass urine.

How many erections a day is normal?

It is different for everyone and it depends on what your hormones are doing too!

EXTRA INFO: You usually get erections because of sexual thoughts and feelings but during puberty, males can get lots of spontaneous erections, i.e. erections that happen for no apparent reason at all. This can happen to all males.

What is sperm?

Sperm is the male reproductive cell and is needed to make a baby.

What is semen?

Semen is the liquid that carries the sperm.

EXTRA INFO: Semen is sticky, cloudy (not clear) and whitish in colour.

EXTRA INFO: Its job is to keep the sperm healthy.

Do I have sperm?

Most males will one day make sperm when they go through puberty, usually when they are between **12-14** years old.

What does ejaculation mean?

Ejaculation is when semen and sperm come out of the penis.

EXTRA INFO: The fluid comes out in little spurts, anywhere between a teaspoon to a tablespoon in volume.

What does semen look like?

Semen is a whitish fluid. It carries and nourishes the sperm.

EXTRA INFO: Semen is made as the male is ejaculating. The ejaculated sperm are pushed through the ejaculatory duct and fluid from the different glands (seminal vesicles, prostate, and Cowper's gland) are added along the way. Most of the fluid comes from the seminal vesicles and prostate gland.

EXTRA INFO: A typical ejaculate is between a teaspoon and tablespoon of fluid containing at least 30 million sperm.

How old do you have to be to make sperm?

Somewhere between **12** to **14** years of age. It is different for every person, but it is usually after your penis and scrotum have started to grow.

Why does my penis sometimes go small?

Usually, because you are cold. All penises do this.

EXTRA INFO: When people get very cold, their penis and scrotum will shrink up, to keep the penis and testicles warm.

When will I start to make sperm?

Males usually start to make sperm when they are **13** and a half. Some will make it sooner and some will make it later.

Wet dreams

What's a 'wet dream'?

A wet dream is when you ejaculate semen and sperm during your sleep. You will have an exciting or sexy dream, your penis will become erect and you will ejaculate semen and sperm.

This is a normal thing to happen to people. Some people have many, some people, not as many, and some people never have a wet dream.

EXTRA INFO: The proper name for a wet dream is 'nocturnal emission'.

When will I start to have wet dreams?

Wet dreams only happen once your body starts to make semen and sperm.

EXTRA INFO: Females can have wet dreams too.

Do all males get wet dreams?

No, some males never have wet dreams.

When do wet dreams happen?

Wet dreams happen at night time during your sleep.

How often will I have wet dreams?

Everyone is different. Some people have lots, some only have one or two, and some people don't have them at all.

Will I know if I have a wet dream?

Sometimes you might wake up during a wet dream but sometimes you don't know until you wake up with a wet patch on your sheets or pyjamas.

What do I do if I have had a wet dream?

You need to decide what you want to happen in your house! Some people are shyer than others, so it may help to try and work out what they want to do.

That's up to you, what do you think we should do?

You might want to put your pyjamas in the wash basket, or start doing your own washing, or...

Puberty

You will find age-appropriate questions and answers about puberty on page 169.

Periods

You will find age-appropriate questions and answers about periods on page 177.

You can access my FREE sex education course for parents at https://sexedrescue.com/back-to-basics/

13 & 14 YEAR OLDS

Sexual intercourse

If your child starts to ask questions about the different types of sexual behavior, it is usually a good idea to find out why they are asking the question. You could very casually say, 'Why are you asking that?' or, 'Where did you hear that word?'

When talking to kids about sex, you can add a value statement about the situations in which you believe sex should happen, e.g. 'In our family, we believe that you shouldn't have sex until...' (you are married, in a loving and committed relationship, are 16, or whatever it is that you believe in).

What is sexual intercourse?

When two adults like each other a lot, they may want to have sexual intercourse with each other. This means that they may hug, kiss and touch each other's bodies all over. The penis becomes erect and the vagina becomes moist and slippery. This makes it easier for the penis to go into the vagina. The male pushes their penis into the vagina (or the female lets the male push their penis into the vagina), they hold each other close, they move around a bit and it can feel good. After a while, the male almost always ejaculates.

EXTRA INFO: Adults have sexual intercourse because they like the way it feels. Their whole body feels good, not just their genitals.

EXTRA INFO: Sexual intercourse is something very private and should happen with (insert your values).

What is sex?

Sex can be lots of different things, but usually, when you hear people talking about baby-making sex, they are talking about sexual intercourse, i.e. penis in vagina sex.

What is casual sex?

Casual sex with someone that you don't know or aren't in a relationship with is common nowadays. So, make sure you talk about the fact that it does happen, and talk about how you feel about it. Try to have a conversation with your child and talk about what they think, too.

EXTRA INFO: Some people have sex with someone that they don't know very well. It could be a complete stranger, or someone that they have met before.

What is foreplay?

Foreplay is the name for all the other stuff, like cuddling and kissing and touching each other's bodies. The stuff that helps to get you into the mood for sex.

Do you have sex with the foreskin forward or backwards?

Usually backwards. When the penis becomes erect (stiff), the foreskin will automatically start to come backwards (retract is the proper word for it).

EXTRA INFO: With some penises the foreskin doesn't retract easily, which means they'll have sex with the foreskin covering the head of their penis. For some people this can feel uncomfortable, which means they need to see a doctor.

Will I ever want to have sex?

Some kids will experience stronger or weaker sexual feelings than others. Some kids will start to have sexual feelings sooner or later than other kids. Everyone is different.

You probably will one day. During puberty, you will start to think about sex differently. This is because of your hormones.

EXTRA INFO: You might find that you start thinking about someone in a new way. You may think about them a lot, have butterflies in your stomach when you meet and daydream about holding hands with them, hugging and kissing.

Will I have sex one day?

Yes, you probably will have sex one day, but it won't be until you are an adult.

When will I want to have sex?

Kids sometimes struggle to understand why they might ever want to have sex one day. One way to explain this is to talk about our 'sex switch.' That switch doesn't get turned on until puberty. Once the switch is turned on, it slowly starts to rewire your brain so that you see sex as something that you want to do instead of something that is weird or gross.

You won't be interested in having sex until puberty happens. Once your body starts making hormones, you will start to think about sex and people in a different way.

EXTRA INFO: Most couples don't just have sex with a complete stranger. They usually start off by getting to know each other first, then become friends. They usually hold hands, hug, cuddle and kiss before they get to the sex part.

Why do people have sex?

Adults have sex for lots of different reasons. To make babies, to show their love for each other, for fun, because it feels good, or to make you feel closer to each other. Having sex is a natural, normal and healthy part of life.

EXTRA INFO: Having sex with someone can be a very intimate experience to share. You can connect with your partner at the most intimate and knowing level that there is.

EXTRA INFO: A lot of things usually happen before a relationship becomes sexual. The 2 people usually start off being friends first and will hold hands, hug, cuddle and kiss before they get to the sex part.

Does it hurt to have sex?

Not usually, but sometimes it can be uncomfortable.

EXTRA INFO: Your body is designed so that it doesn't usually hurt.

Does sex feel good?

Yes, sex usually does feel good. Nature has made sure that sex is enjoyable so that we will want to have sex, which means that babies are being made.

Is it possible to pee inside someone when you are having sex?

No, that isn't possible. When the penis becomes erect, it puts pressure on the muscle that controls urine, which means that urine can't come out of the penis.

EXTRA INFO: Sometimes, if your bladder isn't empty, you can feel like you need to pee because of the pressure placed on the bladder during sex. When you are getting close to orgasm, sometimes you can also feel like you need to pee. But don't worry; you won't.

What's a lubricant?

Lubricant is something that your body makes naturally so that it is easier for the penis to go into the vagina.

EXTRA INFO: You can also buy lubricant as a gel or liquid, in a tube or bottle, that you can use as well.

What is an orgasm?

An orgasm is a really nice feeling that you can get during sex or when you touch your genitals in a nice way (masturbate). For males, it usually happens when the sperm comes out of the penis. For females, it can happen when the outside of the vulva and/or clitoris is rubbed or during vaginal penetration.

Orgasms usually happen when pleasure builds up through sexual intercourse or masturbation. So, you have to be sexually excited and turned on for an orgasm to happen.

Orgasms feel really, really good and are one of the many good things about sex.

EXTRA INFO: Orgasms don't happen every time you have sexual activity. You can still enjoy sex without an orgasm.

EXTRA INFO: Our bodies want us to reproduce, so nature has helped by making sure that sex can feel really good. An orgasm is one of these good things.

How do you have an orgasm?

Orgasms can happen during sexual intercourse, masturbation and when a male has a wet dream. They don't just happen randomly. They happen because of sexual pleasure. (It doesn't just happen spontaneously, as you are walking down the street.)

Why do orgasms happen?

An orgasm usually happens when pleasure builds up through sexual intercourse or masturbation. So, you have to be sexually excited and turned on for an orgasm to happen.

Orgasms feel really, really good and are one of the many good things about sex.

EXTRA INFO: Orgasms don't happen every time you have sexual activity. You can still enjoy sex without an orgasm.

EXTRA INFO: Our bodies want us to reproduce, so nature has helped by making sure that sex can feel really good. An orgasm is one of these good things.

What's an erection?

An erection is when your penis goes hard and erect.

EXTRA INFO: This happens when you have extra blood going into your penis.

EXTRA INFO: All males have erections, and they will start to have more of them as they get closer to puberty.

What does ejaculation mean?

Ejaculation is when semen, which contains sperm, comes out of the penis.

EXTRA INFO: The fluid comes out in little spurts, about a teaspoon in volume.

What is a virgin?

A virgin is someone who hasn't had sexual intercourse before.

How old do you have to be to have sex?

This answer depends on the law in the country and/or state that you live in. If you are unsure, just google 'legal age for sexual consent in (your state or country).'

The law says that you have to be (the legal age where you live). But in our family, we think that you shouldn't have sex until...'

Other sexual activities

Thanks to the oversexualised world we live in (and the porn that kids are exposed to), kids are hearing not just about baby-making-sex, but about all the other types of sex that can happen. Things like anal and oral sex, sexual fetishes, prostitution, bestiality, group sex, sex toys, B&D, S&M, pole dancing, stripping and more. So, you can find age-appropriate answers for questions about these things on page 122.

Love, attraction and gender identity

will find age-appropriate questions and answers about love and attraction and gender identity on page 108.

Contraception

What is abstinence?

Abstinence is when a person decides to not have sexual intercourse.

EXTRA INFO: It is the only 100% effective form of birth control.

What is contraception?

Contraception is something that you can do to prevent pregnancy.

EXTRA INFO: Contraception can be many different things. It could be a tablet that is taken each day, an injection every few months, an implant that goes into the arm or something that is inside the vagina or uterus.

EXTRA INFO: Women can even have a special operation that will stop them from becoming pregnant. It is called a tubal ligation or a hysterectomy.

If your religion doesn't believe in contraception, you will need to talk about natural methods instead. You could try saying, 'Our religion doesn't believe in contraception. So, to try to prevent pregnancy, we have sex when we are less likely to become pregnant.'

Can males use contraception?

Yes, they can. They can use something that will stop a female from becoming pregnant.

EXTRA INFO: Males can wear a condom to stop their sperm from going into the vagina. (A condom is like a special balloon that fits over the penis.)

EXTRA INFO: By the time you are an adult, there may even be an injection or a tablet that men can take. Some males can have a special operation that will stop their sperm from coming out (vasectomy).

Is there anything that you can take after you have had sex?

Emergency contraception, called the morning-after pill, can be supplied over the counter at pharmacies/chemists in Australia, meaning you don't need to see a Doctor for a prescription. If you live outside of Australia, Google it to find out what the rules are in your country.

Yes, the morning-after pill or emergency contraception can be taken within **72** hours of unprotected sex or a broken condom. The sooner it is taken, the sooner it works.

EXTRA INFO: There is no guarantee that it will always work. So, it is not a good idea to rely on it as your only form of contraception.

What's unprotected sex?

Unprotected sex means having vaginal, anal or oral sex without using a condom. This means that you are at risk for STIs and possibly even pregnancy if you haven't used any contraception.

What are the different types of contraception?

Contraception is rapidly changing. The pill is no longer the first choice, with easier and more effective methods now available for females.

No contraception will work **100%** of the time. It has to be used properly, or the chances of it not working are greater. Some methods are not available in all countries.

Condoms

The male condom covers the penis, collecting the sperm to stop it from going into the vagina.

The female condom covers the vulva and fits loosely into the vagina, collecting the sperm before it can go into the vagina.

Diaphragms

The diaphragm is like an elastic cap that gets pushed into the vagina and covers the cervix. It stops the sperm from getting into the uterus. Some people will use it with a spermicide cream that also kills the sperm.

The pill

The pill is a small tablet that you take every day. It tricks the body into thinking it is already pregnant so that it won't release an egg from the ovaries each month. It also changes the mucus at the entrance to the cervix, the entrance to the uterus, which means that the sperm can't get through into the uterus.

The morning-after pill or emergency contraception

A pill that you can take after having unprotected sex or a broken condom that can stop a pregnancy from happening.

Vaginal ring

An elastic ring that is filled with hormones that sits high in the vagina. It tricks the body into thinking it is already pregnant so that it won't release an egg from the ovaries each month.

Intrauterine devices (IUDs)

A small device (it looks like a tiny anchor) that is placed inside the uterus. It tricks the body into thinking it is already pregnant so that it won't release an egg from the ovaries each month.

Implants

A small, thin, flexible rod (like a matchstick) that is inserted under the skin. It tricks the body into thinking it is already pregnant so that it won't release an egg from the ovaries each month. It also changes the mucus at the entrance to the cervix, the entrance to the uterus, which means that the sperm can't get through into the uterus.

Injections

An injection that tricks the body into thinking it is already pregnant so that it won't release an egg from the ovaries each month.

Patch

A sticky patch that is put onto your skin. It tricks the body into thinking it is already pregnant so that it won't release an egg from the ovaries each month. It also changes the mucus at the entrance to the cervix, the entrance to the uterus, which means that the sperm can't get through into the uterus.

What is a condom?

A condom is like a long, skinny balloon, and it covers the penis.

How well do condoms work?

If they are used properly, condoms can work really well.

Can you get condoms for females?

Yes, you can. There are more expensive and are not as easy to find in shops as the male condom.

EXTRA INFO: A female condom is like a big piece of plastic that covers the outside of the vulva, with a long tube bit that gets pushed into the vagina.

What is a vasectomy?

A special operation for males where the tube that carries the sperm from the testicles is cut and tied up so that no sperm can come out. Semen will still come out, but there will be no sperm in it.

EXTRA INFO: The person will still make sperm, but they will just get absorbed into their body.

What is a tubal ligation?

A special operation for females where the tube that carries the egg is cut and tied so that the egg can't come out.

EXTRA INFO: The female will still release an egg each month, but it will just get absorbed into their body.

What is an abortion?

An abortion (or termination) is when a female is pregnant and chooses to have the pregnancy stopped.

They might do this because there is something wrong with them or the baby, or because they don't want to have a baby.

EXTRA INFO: They might have a special operation or take medicine that will make the pregnancy terminate (or finish).

If you are against terminating a pregnancy, you need to tell your child and explain why, e.g. 'I don't believe that people should have abortions because...'

Sexually Transmitted Infections (or STIs)

STIs (sexually transmitted infections) is the current term that we use to describe the things that you can catch when having sex.

When talking about STIs, make sure that you also talk about your family values and religious beliefs in regards to when it is okay for your child to start having sex. It is important to keep on talking about what sexual behaviors and attitudes are okay and not okay in your family, so that your child knows what is expected.

What is an STI?

If someone has germs or viruses in their vagina, penis or blood, they can pass the germs on to the person that they are having sex with. This means that the person that they are having sex with can get sick too.

EXTRA INFO: Some STIs can last a lifetime. Most STIs are treatable, but some aren't.

What are the different types of STIs?

These are the most common STIs. There are other ones as well that are not as common.

There are many different types of STIs. Some are easier to catch than others. Some can be treated, while others can last a lifetime. Some are more common than others.

There are bacterial STIs, like chlamydia, gonorrhoea, and syphilis. These can be treated, but can sometimes cause long-term damage if left untreated.

There are viral STIs, like genital warts, genital herpes, hepatitis and HIV/AIDS. There is no treatment that will get rid of these viruses, but the symptoms can be treated.

Then there are the parasitic STIs, like scabies and crabs. These can be treated with skin washes and shampoos.

What is safe sex?

Safe sex means ways of having sex without getting any infections or becoming pregnant.

EXTRA INFO: It can mean a way to have sex where you don't get semen or vaginal fluid onto the other person's body.

EXTRA INFO: Condoms are one way of having safe sex.

How does the infection spread?

Through skin to skin contact, or through bodily fluids like semen and vaginal secretions. You can't always tell if someone has an STI just by looking.

EXTRA INFO: Every infection is different. Some are spread easily, while others are harder to spread.

EXTRA INFO: Some viruses are also spread from blood, like HIV and Hepatitis B and C.

How will I know if I have a STI?

You might have a discharge from your vagina or penis, or find sores, redness, a rash or irritation in the genital area; it might hurt to have sex, or burn when you pass urine.

EXTRA INFO: Sometimes you may not know that you have an STI. This means that you can infect other people without even knowing.

How do you prevent STIs?

You might use a condom, which will stop any infections from getting inside your penis or vagina. A condom will prevent most STIs, but not all.

EXTRA INFO: Once you start having sex, you can also start having STI checks, which is where they test you for any infections that you may have caught through sexual contact.

How well do condoms work at preventing STIs?

Condoms are not **100%** effective. If used properly, they can do a pretty good job, but some infections can still be spread.

What's unprotected sex?

Unprotected sex means having vaginal, anal or oral sex without using a condom. This means that you are at risk for STIs and possibly even pregnancy if you haven't used any contraception.

What happens if a condom falls off in the vagina?

It is pretty uncommon for this to happen, but if it happens, it means that they may be at risk for pregnancy and/or catching an STI.

EXTRA INFO: Once the male has ejaculated, the penis will shrink, which means that the condom can be left behind if they don't hold on to the condom when they withdraw their penis.

Can you use a condom more than once?

No, you can't. Condoms are only meant to be used once. Plus, there is a very good chance that the condom would break if you reused it. This would mean that you could become pregnant or catch an STI.

Can you use a balloon, or something else like a plastic bag, if you don't have a condom?

No, you should never try to use something else. Anything else would break and may not block any STIs or sperm from coming through whatever it is that you are using.

What happens if the condom doesn't work, or it breaks?

If the condom isn't put on properly, or if it breaks, there is a much greater chance of pregnancy or catching an STI.

Where do you buy condoms from?

Nowadays, you can buy them almost anywhere. Supermarkets, pharmacies, and convenience stores carry them. Some public restrooms have machines on their walls that sell them. You can even buy them online.

What's AIDS?

AIDS is the name of a disease. It is caused by a virus called HIV (Human Immunodeficiency Virus).

EXTRA INFO: A virus is like a germ, in that it can make people get very sick.

EXTRA INFO: Sometimes you hear people talking about AIDS. When it first came out, a lot of people died from it, and because it was spread through sex and blood, a lot of people were scared.

How do people get AIDS?

They either need to have sexual intercourse with that person or share blood with them, like if you used someone else's drug needle after they had used it.

Can only gay people get AIDS?

No, anyone can get the HIV virus if they come in contact with it. When we first learned about HIV and AIDS, everyone thought it was a gay disease because it was affecting so many gay males. But we soon realized that it was affecting other people as well.

What is herpes?

Herpes is the name of a virus that can cause cold sores (blisters) on the mouth and the genitals. If someone has a cold sore on their mouth, and they put their mouth on your penis or vulva, you could end up with cold sores on your genitals. This is called genital herpes, and it is an STI.

What are genital warts?

A wart in the genital area is caused by the Human Papilloma Virus (HPV), which is an STI. It is spread through sexual contact and can leave warts on the genitals.

EXTRA INFO: Some strains of HPV cause cancer. There is now a vaccine that prevents HPV for young adults.

What is cervical cancer?

Cervical cancer is cancer that happens in the cervix (the opening of the uterus).

EXTRA INFO: HPV is responsible for more than 70% of cervical cancers. There is now a vaccine out that prevents HPV in young adults, and now we are seeing a lot less cervical cancer in young women.

What is a pap smear or cervical screening test?

The frequency of cervical screening is changing and varies from country to country. In some countries, it is every 2 or 4 years. Since the introduction of the HPV vaccine, the frequency of screening is changing.

A pap smear test or cervical screening is a screening test for females that they need to have every few years. They can be embarrassing (because someone has to look at your vulva), but they are very important.

EXTRA INFO: You need to go to see a doctor or nurse to have this done. They will ask you to take off your underpants, and then you lie down on your back, on a special bed, with a sheet on top of you. You have to open up your legs, and they put a plastic speculum into your vagina. This allows them to see your cervix, which is at the very end of your vagina. They then use a small brush, which they gently rub over the cervix, to collect the cervical cells and place them onto a glass slide. The slide then goes to a special laboratory, where they look and see if there are any unusual cells that could be cancerous.

Penises and erections

Don't forget to remind your child that we all start puberty at different times. And that our bodies will all change differently. Breasts, penises and our bodies come in all different shapes and sizes. Reassure them that they are normal.

What is an erection?

An erection is when the amount of blood going to the penis increases, making the penis hard and erect.

EXTRA INFO: An erect penis is much bigger than a soft one and stands away from the body.

EXTRA INFO: All males have erections but during puberty, they happen more often.

EXTRA INFO: Sometimes erections happen for no reason at all. You don't have to be sexually aroused to have an erection.

Why do I have erections?

All males have erections, and even little kids and babies get them too.

They can happen when you are having sexy thoughts when the penis is touched or rubbed by clothing. Sometimes they can happen for no reason at all.

Can I stop myself from having an erection?

During puberty, erections can sometimes happen for no reason at all. It can be very embarrassing for people when this happens.

EXTRA INFO: Unwanted erections will go away more quickly if you think of something else (like saying the alphabet backwards).

EXTRA INFO: Unwanted erections won't happen forever. Once puberty is over, you will find that you have more control over your erections.

Why do I wake up with an erection?

It is common for people to wake up with an erection. They usually happen during the REM (Rapid Eye Movement) phase of sleep, which is just before you wake up. Sometimes it can also be because you have a full bladder.

EXTRA INFO: If you happen to have a sexy dream during this phase, you will sometimes ejaculate.

EXTRA INFO: A full bladder can place pressure on the erectile tissue at the base of the penis, causing an erection. Because you can't wee with an erection, you will have to wait a few minutes for your penis to relax before you can pass urine.

How many erections a day is normal?

It is different for everyone and it depends on what your hormones are doing too!

EXTRA INFO: You usually get erections because of sexual thoughts and feelings but during puberty, males can get lots of spontaneous erections, i.e. erections that happen for no apparent reason at all. This can happen to all males.

What is sperm?

Sperm are the male sex cells, i.e. the male part that you need to join with the female ovum (or egg) to make a baby.

EXTRA INFO: Sperm is made in the testicles. They take about 2 weeks to be fully grown and are then stored in the epididymis, where they are either ejaculated out or absorbed back into the body, 4-5 weeks later.

What is semen?

Semen is the liquid that carries the sperm.

EXTRA INFO: Semen is sticky, cloudy (not clear) and whitish in colour.

EXTRA INFO: Its job is to keep the sperm healthy.

What's the difference between sperm and semen?

Sperm is made by your testicles during puberty and is needed to make a baby. Semen is the whitish fluid that carries the sperm.

Do I have sperm?

Most males will one day make sperm when they go through puberty, usually when they are between 12-14 years old.

When will I start to make sperm?

Males usually start to make sperm when they are 13 and a half. Some will make it sooner and some will make it later.

What does ejaculation mean?

Ejaculation is when semen and sperm come out of the penis.

EXTRA INFO: The fluid comes out in little spurts, anywhere between a teaspoon to a tablespoon in volume.

What does semen look like?

Semen is a whitish fluid. It carries and nourishes the sperm.

EXTRA INFO: Semen is made as the male is ejaculating. The ejaculated sperm are pushed through the ejaculatory duct and fluid from the different glands (seminal vesicles, prostate, and Cowper's gland) are added along the way. Most of the fluid comes from the seminal vesicles and prostate gland.

EXTRA INFO: A typical ejaculate is between a teaspoon and tablespoon of fluid containing at least 30 million sperm.

How old do you have to be to make sperm?

Somewhere between **12** to **14** years of age. It is different for every person, but it is usually after your penis and scrotum have started to grow.

How does sperm come out?

Semen joins the sperm and this liquid is pushed out through the penis during muscular contractions, i.e. orgasm. This can happen during masturbation, a wet dream or during sexual activity.

The sperm comes out with each muscular contraction, in small spurts or dribbles.

EXTRA INFO: The fastest speed recorded is 40 km/hour (or 25 miles/hour).

Will I run out of sperm?

No, your body makes sperm throughout your whole life.

My penis is growing longer, is that normal?

Yes, they do that during puberty. They grow longer and then they grow wider.

Why is one of my testicles bigger than the other?

Sometimes this is just what happens. Testicles are often different in size and one may hang a little lower than the other one. This also stops them from knocking against each other.

Is it normal for my penis to bend?

Sometimes the penis can have a slight bend to it, especially when it is erect.

What happens if your foreskin can't push back?

When the penis is erect, the foreskin will automatically pull back by its self. Sometimes you might need to help push it back, to have it pulled back all the way.

EXTRA INFO: If the foreskin is too tight to push back, or if it hurts or is uncomfortable when it is pushed back, you will need to see a Doctor. This is not uncommon and happens to other people too.

Why does my penis sometimes go small?

Usually, because you are cold. All penises do this.

EXTRA INFO: When males get very cold, their penis and scrotum will shrink up, to keep the penis and testicles warm.

Wet dreams

What's a 'wet dream'?

A wet dream is when you ejaculate semen and sperm during your sleep. You will have an exciting or sexy dream, your penis will become erect and you will ejaculate semen and sperm.

This is a normal thing to happen to people. Some people have many, some people, not as many and some people never have a wet dream.

EXTRA INFO: The proper name for a wet dream is 'nocturnal emission'.

When will I start to have wet dreams?

Wet dreams only happen once your body starts to make semen and sperm.

Do all males get wet dreams?

No, some males never have wet dreams.

Why do males have wet dreams?

Wet dreams help a male's body to get rid of the extra sperm that they produce.

EXTRA INFO: It is common for males to experience an erection during the REM (Rapid Eye Movement) phase of sleep, which is the phase just before you wake up. If you happen to have a sexy dream during this phase, you will sometimes ejaculate.

When do wet dreams happen?

Wet dreams happen at night time during your sleep.

How often will I have wet dreams?

Everyone is different. Some people have lots, some only have one or two, and some people don't have them at all.

Will I know if I have a wet dream?

Sometimes you might wake up during a wet dream but sometimes you don't know until you wake up with a wet patch on your sheets or pyjamas.

What do I do if I have a wet dream?

You need to decide what you want to happen in your house! Some people are shyer than others, so it may help to try and work out what they want to do.

That's up to you: what do you think we should do?

You might want to put your pyjamas in the wash basket, or start doing your own washing, or...

Puberty

You will find age-appropriate questions and answers about puberty on page 169.

Periods

You will find age-appropriate questions and answers about periods on page 177.

 You can access my FREE sex education course for parents at https://sexedrescue.com/back-to-basics/

RESOURCES

If you are looking for a list of resources on sex education, then you won't find that in this book.

Why? Because by the time you have gotten around to reading this book, the list will already be out of date!

So instead of providing you with a list that is already out of date, I'll tell you about some online resources that I update regularly whenever I find some new content, discover a new website, read a new journal article or blogpost, or buy a newly published book.

So...

- To get started with sex education, sign up for my FREE sex education course for parents: https://sexedrescue.com/back-to-basics/
- To find a list of all the wonderful content that is available on the internet on sex education, you can go to: https://sexedrescue.com/sex-education-resources/
- To find a comprehensive list of sex education books for your child to read, you can go to: https://sexedrescue.com/sex-education-books-for-children/
- To ask questions about sex education and to connect with other parents on the same journey, you can join my free parent Facebook group: https://www.facebook.com/groups/thatparentgroup/
- To receive regular information about sex education, you can sign up for my newsletter: https://sexedrescue.com/newsletter/

- Plus, you will find videos, articles and lots of other educational content at Sex Ed Rescue: https://sexedrescue.com

REFERENCES

An Overview of Child Development Theories by Angela Oswalt. Mental Health Services of Southern Carolina. Accessed 6 October 2017 http:// www.mhsso. org/poc/view_doc.php?type=doc&id=7918&cn=28

Child Sexual Development by Loretta Haroian. Electronic Journal of Human Sexuality, Volume 3. Accessed 6 October 2017 http://www.ejhs.org/volume3/ Haroian/body.htm

Children's Sexual Development and Behaviour – Pants aren't Rude (second edition) by Pam Linke. 2015. Early Childhood Australia.

Flight of the Stork: What Children Think (and When) about Sex and Family Building by Anne C. Bernstein. 1994. Perspectives press. Indianapolis.

Handbook of Child and Adolescent Sexuality: Developmental and Forensic Psychology. Edited by Daniel S. Bromberg and William T. O'Donohue. 2013. Elsevier. Academic Press. Oxford.

Information by Age. Alberta Health Services. Accessed 6 October 2017. https:// teachingsexualhealth.ca/parents/information-by-age/

Is This Normal? Understanding Your Child's Sexual Behaviors by Holly Brennan and Judy Graham. 2012. Family Planning Queensland. Fortitude Valley.

Show me Yours! Understanding Children's Sexuality by Ronald and Juliette Goldman. 1988. Penguin Books Australia. Ringwood.

Understanding Your Child's Sexual Behaviour: What's Natural and Healthy by Toni Cavanagh Johnson. 1999. New Harbinger Publications, Inc. Oakland.

Where do I start? *Supporting Healthy Sexual Development in Early Childhood* by Family Planning Queensland. 2009. Family Planning Queensland. Fortitude Valley.

ABOUT THE AUTHOR

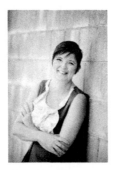

Ca th Hakanson has been talking to clients about sex for the past 25 years as a nurse, midwife, sex therapist, researcher, author and educator. She's spent the past 11 years trying to unravel why parents (herself included) struggle with sex education. Her solution was to create Sex Ed Rescue, an online resource that simplifi es sex education and helps parents to empower their children with the right information about sex, so kids can talk to them about anything, no matter what.

Cath has lived all over Australia but currently lives in Perth with her partner, 2 children, and ever-growing menagerie of pets. Despite having an unusual profession, she bakes, sews, and knits for sanity, collects sexual trivia, and tries really hard not to embarrass her children in public. Well, most of the time anyway!

If you'd like to know more, please visit her online home at SexEdRescue.com

Printed in Great Britain
by Amazon

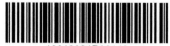